Thromboembolism:
Diagnosis and Treatment

Thromboembolism: Diagnosis and Treatment

THE PROCEEDINGS OF A SYMPOSIUM HELD AT
KING'S COLLEGE HOSPITAL, LONDON
SPONSORED BY KABI PHARMACEUTICALS LIMITED

Editors

V. V. KAKKAR, F.R.C.S.E., F.R.C.S.
Senior Lecturer in Surgery,
King's College Hospital Medical School, London

A. J. JOUHAR, M.B., M.R.C.S.
Medical Director, Kabi Pharmaceuticals Limited,
Ealing, London.

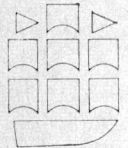

The Williams & Wilkins Company
Baltimore

First Published 1972

ISBN 0 443 00919 8

© Longman Group Ltd. 1972

All rights reserved. No part of this publication may be reproduced, stored in a retrieval system, or transmitted, in any form or by any means, electronic, mechanical, photo-copying, recording or otherwise, without the prior permission of the copyright owner.

Any correspondence relating to this volume should be directed to the publishers at 104 Gloucester Place, London W1H 4AE.

*Printed in Great Britain by
The Whitefriars Press Ltd, London and Tonbridge*

Foreword

The Rt. Hon. Lord Brock, M.S., F.R.C.S.
Director, Department of Surgical Sciences,
Royal College of Surgeons of England

Venous thromboembolism has for many years been the Cinderella of clinical medicine and surgery. What interest there has been is largely due to its importance in relation to operations and surgical conditions, but it is now fully recognised that it is equally responsible for disability and death in medical as well as surgical cases. Much of the approach to this problem in surgical cases has been empirical and hence not constructive. Medical interest has been even less.

During recent years more attention has been paid to the problem and it has been studied in a methodical and scientific manner. Notable advances have been made in treatment as a result of this new knowledge. These advances have been in prevention, clearly the most acceptable, and treatment of the thrombotic process with more success achieved in the treatment of pulmonary embolism. This has not only been in the actual safety of pulmonary embolectomy but also in its management by non-operative thrombolytic means.

This symposium was a planned attempt to get together all the new knowledge and by presentation and discussion to consolidate this knowledge to the benefit of all. The printing and publication of the symposium gives a permanent record and enables everyone to share the large volume of valuable information and experience that was presented.

It will be found that every aspect is dealt with. The altered physiological states, especially in relation to hypercoagulability, the anatomical factors and the dynamic changes of thrombosis as opposed to vague assumption. The important factors of prevention are presented and also reversal of the thrombotic state by thrombolytic therapy.

Surgical treatment of the established state is almost obligatory if the years of severe and increasing disability from the damaged venous system of the lower limbs is to be avoided or mitigated. Lastly the management of established pulmonary embolism is fully dealt with.

This is a book that can help everybody, medical or surgical, senior or junior. I wish it the success it deserves.

Preface

Fortunate indeed are those who are involved in the study of thrombosis. There have been spectacular advances over the last few years. Insight into the process and how it may be modified has arisen from work in the laboratories. But the main spur to recent understanding, particularly with regard to thromboembolism, has been the introduction of sensitive and precise methods for measuring thrombosis in patients. Now we can observe the process as it actually occurs, whether it is increasing or decreasing in extent or remaining stationary. Now we can measure with great accuracy the efficacy of attempts to prevent deep vein thrombosis following operation and to treat the condition. With such tools we have every right to expect great advances in the management of thromboembolism in the near future. The timing of this Symposium on the subject is most propitious.

The idea for the Conference, which was held on July 10th 1971, came from Mr. V. V. Kakkar. Without his drive and effort the venture would not have been possible. I think that some measure of his prowess in the field is reflected by the many and distinguished participants from all parts of the world who were persuaded to take part in the meeting.

All of us are indebted to Kabi Pharmaceuticals Limited for responding so generously to our request for financial support for the Symposium and the publication of the Proceedings.

I would like to express our gratitude to Lord Brock, London, Professor Sol Sherry, Philadelphia, Dr. A. A. Sharp, Oxford and Mr. C. T. Howe, King's College Hospital, London, for chairing various sessions.

I also wish to thank Mrs. M. G. Shelton and Mrs. M. Morrison for their help in organising the Symposium and dealing with the manuscripts, and Miss J. Davidson for the final typescript of this publication.

London 1972   J. G. MURRAY
Professor of Surgery, King's College Hospital.

Contents

Foreword v

Preface J. G. Murray vii

Contributors xi

PART I: PRINCIPLES OF THROMBOEMBOLISM

1. The blood and venous thromboembolism . . . 2
   P. T. Flute, V. V. Kakkar, J. T. G. Renney and A. N. Nicolaides

2. The issue of hypercoagulability 13
   S. Wessler

3. Fibrinogen-fibrin degradation products and venous thromboembolism 25
   A. P. Fletcher, N. Alkjaersig and J. O'Brien

4. New laboratory tests for the diagnosis of venous thromboembolism 39
   V. Gurewich

5. Discussion to Part 1. 49

PART II: PREVENTION AND DIAGNOSIS

6. The dynamics of venous blood flow and the prevention of deep venous thrombosis 56
   L. T. Cotton, S. Sabri and V. C. Roberts

7. Soleal veins, stasis and prevention of deep vein thrombosis 69
   A. N. Nicolaides, V. V. Kakkar, E. S. Field and P. Fish

8. Diagnosis of deep venous thrombosis and its sequelae by Doppler ultrasound detection 89
   B. Sigel, W. R. Felix, Jr., J. Ipsen and G. L. Popky

9. Isotopic detection of deep venous thrombosis . . 101
   V. V. Kakkar

10. Deep vein thrombosis after myocardial infarction, prostatectomy and fracture of the femoral neck . . . 117
    E. S. Field, V. V. Kakkar and A. N. Nicolaides

11. Deep vein thrombosis in obstetric and gynaecological patients 131
    J. R. Friend and V. V. Kakkar

12. Discussion to Part 2 139

PART III: MEDICAL TREATMENT

13. Is thrombolytic therapy justified? 144
    S. Sherry

14. Drug therapy of venous thromboembolism . . . 155
    D. P. Thomas

15. Treatment of deep vein thrombosis with streptokinase . 169
    V. V. Kakkar and P. T. Flute

16. Streptokinase and pulmonary embolism . . . 181
    G. C. Sutton, G. A. H. Miller, I. H. Kerr,
    R. V. Gibson and M. Honey

17. NHLI urokinase pulmonary embolism trial: Phase I results of a controlled study 195
    A. A. Sasahara, J. S. Belko, G. V. R. K. Sharma,
    K. M. McIntyre, R. L. Morse and T. M. Hyers

PART IV: SURGICAL TREATMENT

18. Embolectomy and pulmonary embolism: criteria for surgery 212
    P. A. Cullum, V. V. Kakkar, A. M. Macarthur and E. B. Raftery

19. Surgical treatment of pulmonary embolism . . . 223
    M. Paneth

20. Discussions to Parts 3 and 4 229

    Index 235

Contributors

L. T. Cotton, M.Ch., F.R.C.S.	Consultant Surgeon, King's College Hospital, London.
P. A. Cullum, F.R.C.S.	Senior Lecturer in Cardiothoracic Surgery and Honorary Consultant, King's College Hospital Medical School, London.
E. S. Field, F.R.C.S.	Research Fellow, King's College Hospital Medical School, London.
A. P. Fletcher, M.D.	Professor of Medicine, Washington University, St. Louis, Missouri, U.S.A.
P. T. Flute, M.D., M.R.C.Path.	Reader in Haematology, King's College Hospital Medical School, London.
J. R. Friend, M.A., M.R.C.O.G.	Senior Registrar Obstetric Gynaecology, King's College Hospital Medical School, London.
V. Gurewich, M.D.	Assistant Clinical Professor of Medicine, Harvard Medical School, Boston, Massachusetts, U.S.A.
V. V. Kakkar, F.R.C.S.E., F.R.C.S.	Senior Lecturer in Surgery, King's College Hospital Medical School, London.
A. N. Nicolaides, F.R.C.S.E., F.R.C.S.	Surgical Unit, St. Mary's Hospital, London.
M. Paneth, F.R.C.S.	Thoracic Surgeon, Brompton Hospital, London.
A. A. Sasahara, M.D.	Director, Cardiopulmonary Laboratory, V.A. Hospital, West Roxbury, Massachusetts, U.S.A.
S. Sherry, M.D.	Professor of Medicine, Temple University, Philadelphia, Pennsylvania, U.S.A.

B. Sigel, M.D.	Professor of Surgery, Medical College of Pennsylvania, U.S.A.
G. C. Sutton, M.R.C.P.	Senior Registrar in Cardiology, Brompton Hospital, London.
D. P. Thomas, M.D., B.Sc., D.Phil.	Department of Pharmacology, Royal College of Surgeons of England, London.
S. Wessler, M.D.	Professor of Medicine, Washington University, St. Louis, Missouri, U.S.A.

PART I
PRINCIPLES OF THROMBOEMBOLISM

1 The Blood and Venous Thromboembolism

P. T. Flute, V. V. Kakkar, J. T. G. Renney and A. N. Nicolaides

There is, at present, no laboratory test which will allow the recognition of incipient or actual thrombosis. However, a major difficulty in investigating the significance of blood changes in this respect has been resolved now that the ^{125}I-fibrinogen test (Kakkar et al., 1970a) is available as a means of diagnosis. This test provides for the first time an absolute means by which to discriminate between those patients who have a thrombus in the deep calf veins and those who have not. Since the great majority of thrombi arise in this situation (Kakkar et al., 1970b) laboratory results can be analysed with some confidence that they are being allocated to the correct group, to see whether any particular change is characteristic of thrombosis.

So many interacting factors contribute to the formation of a thrombus that it is, perhaps, impossible to expect a precise dividing line between the patient who is at high risk of developing a thrombus and one in whom actual deposition of fibrin has already occurred within major veins. Some degree of stimulation of intravascular coagulation is probably a common event in many diseases. The stimulus might come directly from damaged vessel walls or indirectly from entry into the blood of potentially coagulant materials from inflamed tissue. While blood flow continues the active coagulation enzymes will be carried away from the site of a local stimulus to be cleared into cells of the reticulo-enthothelial system (Wessler et al., 1967) and while in transit their effect will be held in check by inhibitors in the plasma, which are capable of neutralising more of the enzyme than can possibly be generated from the unit volume of blood in which they are contained. These important inhibitors include antithrombin III, which recently has been shown to have even greater inhibitory power against activated factor X (factor Xa) (Yin et al., 1971). Thrombosis is likely when these compensating mechanisms are overwhelmed, particularly so in areas of reduced blood flow (Wessler and Yin, 1968). There is no direct way in which to recognise the presence in the blood of active coagulation factors, which are not differentiated from their inactive precursors by the usual assay systems. However, their presence sometimes has been inferred from their effects in states where the blood contains soluble fibrin monomer complexes (Kowalski, 1968) or fibrin/fibrinogen degradation products (FDP) of fibrinolysis (Merskey et al., 1966).

The increased risk of thrombosis after surgical operation is well recognised and this period has been used for detailed investigation on many occasions. The true incidence of post-operative thrombosis in the deep calf veins is now known to be between 20 and 30 per cent of patients, with an even higher incidence in older patients undergoing major operations (Kakkar et al., 1970b). The effects of severe blood loss on the coagulation time are easy to appreciate. William Hewson in 1772, observing the killing of sheep, noted that 'the blood which issued last coagulated first'. Detailed investigations of the effects of blood loss and trauma which appear to stimulate coagulation and fibrinolysis have been reported in experimental animals (Bergentz and Nilsson, 1961; Penick et al., 1965; Hardaway, 1967; Leandoer, 1968), in injured patients (Innes and Sevitt, 1964), and after surgery (Egeberg, 1962; Phillips et al., 1963; Flute, 1965; Barkhan, 1969; Ygge, 1970). After surgery there is an increase of the platelet count (Sharnoff et al., 1960), sometimes after an initial fall; platelet adhesiveness is also increased (Wright, 1942; Bennet, 1967; Ham and Slack, 1967). After an initial fall, which is not always detectable, the concentration of many coagulation factors increases in the blood (Davidson and Tomlin, 1963). The increase is particularly obvious for fibrinogen (Godal, 1962) and factor VIII (Amundsen et al., 1963; Penick et al., 1965; Penick et al., 1966). There is an increased heparin tolerance (Gormson and Haxholdt, 1960) and decreased heparin co-factor activity (Olsson, 1963; Olsson et al., 1964). Spontaneous fibrinolytic activity of the blood due to circulating plasminogen activator is increased at first, but subsequently falls (Innes and Sevitt, 1964; Flute, 1965; Pison et al., 1965; Leandoer, 1968). Plasminogen is decreased (Flute, 1965) and later may increase (Ygge, 1970). FDP appear in the serum (Cash et al., 1969; Borowiecki and Sharp, 1969; Prentice et al., 1969; Ruckley et al., 1970) and there is an increased precipitation when plasma is mixed with protamine, which suggests the presence of circulating fibrin monomer complexes (Lipinski and Worowski, 1968). Recent studies have shown an increase in both the fractional catabolic rate and the absolute catabolism of fibrinogen in the period after operation (Atkins and Hawkins, 1969; Lim et al., 1969;

Davies et al., 1970; Hickman, 1971). These changes could all be interpreted as evidence for the stimulation of coagulation and fibrinolysis. The initial falls would then be due to increased consumption of the available factors and the subsequent increases as overproduction in response to the sudden demand (McKay, 1969; Flute, 1970; Hardaway, 1970).

A selection from these possible changes was made and serial tests carried out in patients undergoing surgery who were screened for the presence of thrombi by careful clinical examination, the ^{125}I-fibrinogen test and, in a few cases, by phlebography. The study to correlate blood changes with the incidence of thrombosis is still in progress, but preliminary results are available.

METHODS

Blood samples were collected into potassium sequestrene (1 mg) of blood for platelet count; and into one tenth volume of 3·8 per cent trisodium citrate in polystyrene containers, previously cooled in a bath of melting ice, for coagulation and fibrinolysis studies. Venepuncture samples were obtained on the day before operation and on the first, second, third and sixth post-operative days.

Platelet counts were performed by the method of Brecher and Cronkite (1950).

Platelet adhesiveness was determined by the method of Hellem (1960; 1968). Citrated blood was passed at constant speed through a 9 cm length of Portex NT10 soft transparent tubing packed with 1 g of Jencon's No. 8 glass ballotini.

Plasma fibrinogen was measured by the clot weight method of Ingram (1961). Two ml of citrated plasma was clotted with 2 ml of 0·025M calcium chloride containing 10 NIH units of thrombin (Thrombin Topical, Parke Davis Limited) and 20 mg of tranexamic acid (Cyklokapron, Kabi Pharmaceuticals Limited). The clot which formed after 30 minutes at 37°C was wound onto a wooden applicator stick, washed in distilled water, cut from the stick, dried first in acetone for 10 minutes and then at 37°C for 24 hours before being weighed. The results are expressed as mg per 100 ml of citrated plasma.

Dilute clot lysis time was obtained according to Fearnley et al. (1957). The initial tenfold dilutions of blood were set up immediately after venepuncture, kept in glass tubes in an ice bath for 30 minutes and then incubated at 37°C. For analysis the results have been divided into arbitrary groups of those with lysis times of less than 2 hours (group 1, very high activator concentration), 2 to 7 hours (group 2, average activator concentration), 7 to 24 hours (group 3, low activator concentration) and over 24 hours (group 4, very low activator concentration). This method has been adopted because the exponential relationship between lysis time and activator concentration makes the direct comparison of actual lysis times difficult. In addition, changes in fibrinogen concentration could have contributed to minor differences in lysis time, but they are unlikely to have a significant effect on such widely spaced groups.

Serum FDP (fibrinogen/fibrin degradation products) were measured by the human tanned red cell haemagglutination inhibition technique of Merskey *et al.* (1969). Estimations were performed using the supernatant from the fibrinogen estimation, from which the fibrin had been removed. The anti-fibrinogen serum was obtained from Behringwerke. Standards were set up with each batch of tests, using the plasma and the fibrinogen supernate from the same healthy individual. Pre-operative values were always less than 2 μg per ml.

Protamine precipitation was measured by the method of Lipinski and Worowski (1968). Light transmission 5 minutes after the addition of protamine to citrated plasma was measured in a 1 cm cell in an EEL model A colorimeter, using an Ilford 608 filter.

In vivo scanning after the injection of ^{125}I-*labelled fibrinogen* was performed as described by Flanc *et al.* (1969).

Analysis of the results: All the haematological results and important clinical data were analysed by a PDP 8 computer programme. The daily mean and the standard deviation of the mean were calculated for the result of each test for the patient population as a whole and also for selected groups of the patients, for example, those with deep vein thrombosis, and those without. Thus, it was possible to compare each day's mean with the pre-operative mean for the same test and also to compare the mean for a particular test in a separate group of the patients with the corresponding mean for any other group on the same day. The significance of any difference was judged by Student's t-test. Finally, the correlation coefficients were calculated between the daily means for the different tests.

SELECTION OF PATIENTS

Ninety-two consecutive general surgical patients over the age of 40 years have been studied. The only patients excluded were those having operations on the legs, which might have prejudiced the results of the ^{125}I-fibrinogen test, those with operations on the thyroid gland, and those with a history of recent deep vein thrombosis before operation. Seventy-four of the patients received infusions of dextran (Macrodex 70, Pharmacia Limited) before and after operation, as part of a trial designed to test the effects of this drug on the incidence of deep vein thrombosis. Full details of this trial, which did not give a dramatic reduction in the incidence of thrombosis in the patients studied, will be given elsewhere. Minor operations, including herniorrhaphy, simple mastectomy, and biopsy of the superficial structures, were performed in 31 of the patients. In the remainder, classified as severe operations, the abdominal cavity was opened.

RESULTS

There were significant increases of fibrinogen, lysis time, serum FDP, and platelet count at various times after operation (Fig. 1.1). These are the changes which would have been expected. Correlation between the change in the mean results for the plasma fibrinogen and the protamine precipitate test were so close (r 0.93, $p < 0.01$) that the latter results have not been presented separately. Changes in fibrinogen and lysis time (r 0.77, $p < 0.05$) and fibrinogen and platelet count (r 0.73, $p < 0.05$) showed rather less close correlation. None of the other results appeared to be significantly related.

The increase which was observed in platelet adhesiveness failed to reach the degree of significance expected from previous studies. The reason for this is apparent when patients receiving dextran are separated from the remainder (Fig. 1.2). Without dextran, platelet adhesiveness and platelet count are increased significantly. The infusion of dextran made no appreciable difference to changes in fibrinogen, lysis time, or FDP.

Within the whole group, thrombi were detected in 39 limbs of 27 patients. When patients with thrombosis are separated from the remainder it is possible to see which of the tests are characteristic of thrombosis. The two groups have been plotted separately in addition to the results for the whole population in Fig. 1.1. The only significant difference is in the result for the lysis time which is slightly longer on the second day in patients with deep vein thrombosis. Little importance can be attached to such an isolated finding. There was no significant difference in fibrinogen nor in FDP despite the inclusion of three patients with undoubted pulmonary embolism in the thrombosis group. These three patients, the only ones in whom pulmonary embolism was recognised, had the highest values for serum FDP—12, 42 and 95 μg per ml respectively. These were found after the onset of symptoms from the embolus and before that they were unremarkable. Differences in platelet count or adhesiveness were not significant, even when patients receiving dextran were considered separately.

Thus the test results correlate with each other, but show no ability to define the patients with deep vein thrombosis. As has been shown by others, the incidence of thrombosis was much greater in those

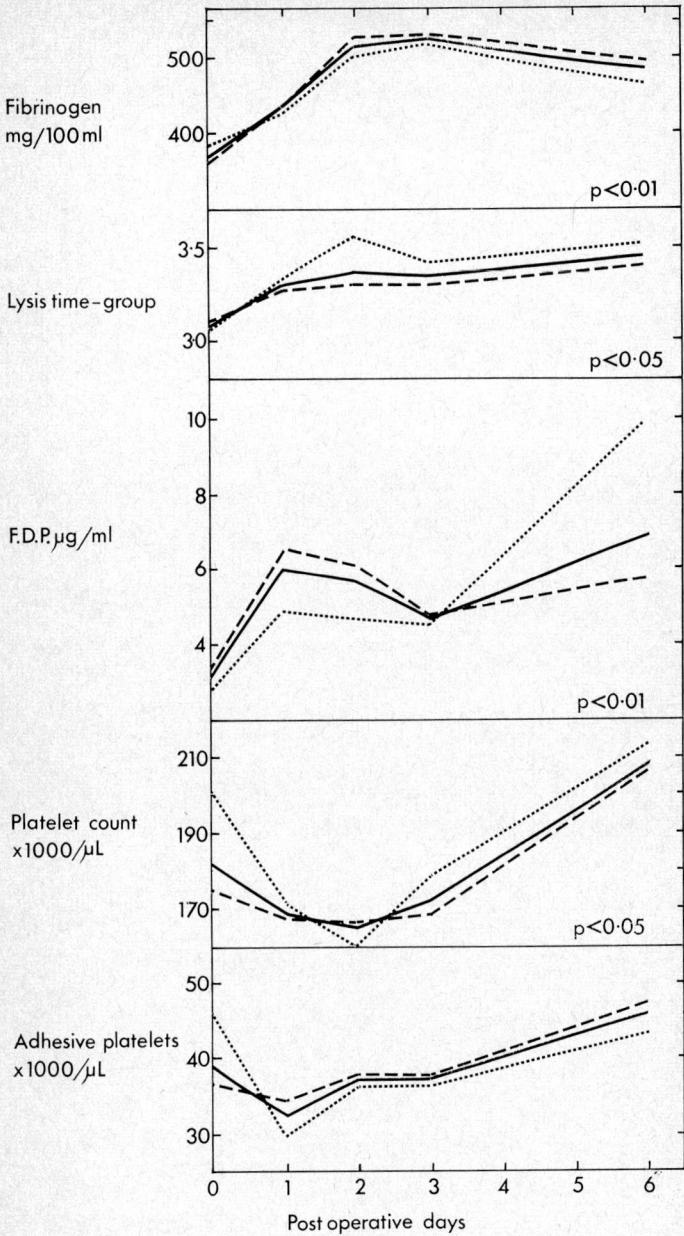

FIG. 1.1. The mean value for each test on a particular day, shown for all 92 patients, and again for the 27 patients who developed thrombosis and the 65 who did not.

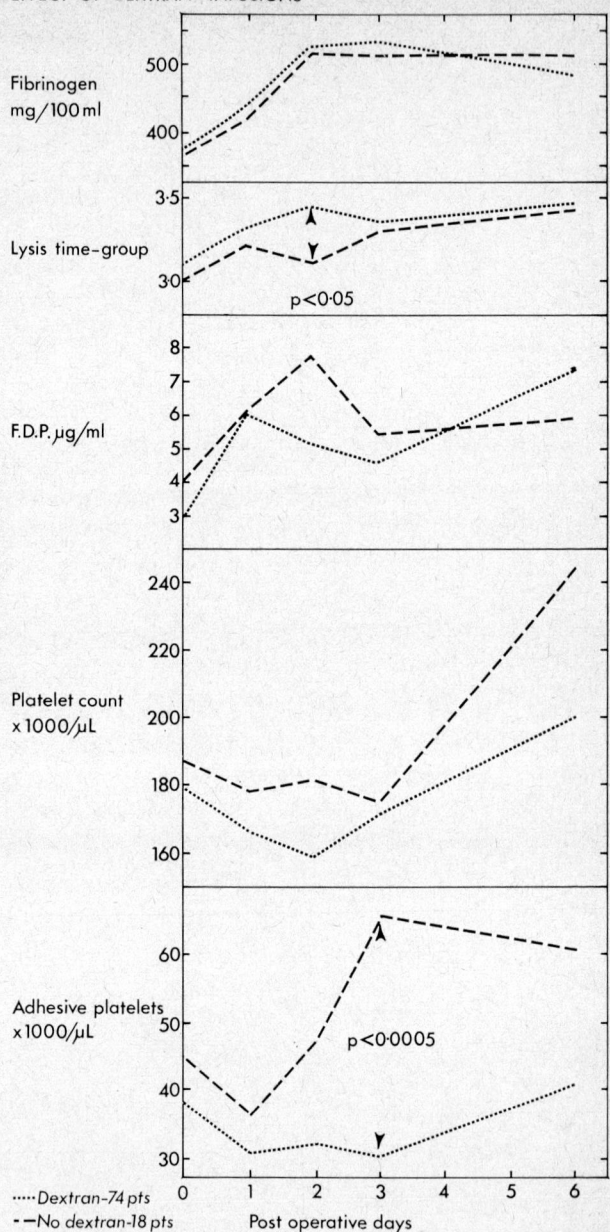

FIG. 1.2. The mean value for each test on a particular day for the 74 patients who received dextran infusions and the 18 patients who did not.

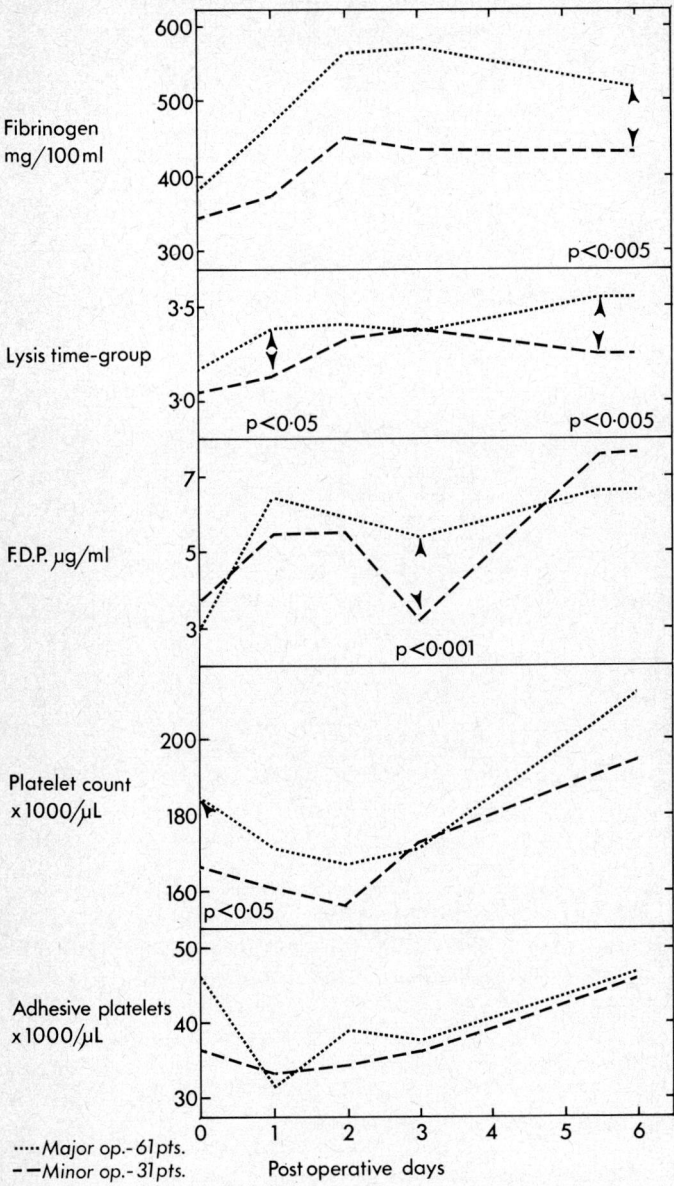

FIG. 1.3. The mean value for each test on a particular day for the 31 patients who had minor operations and the 61 patients who had major operations.

having major rather than minor operations: 36 per cent of the former and 16 per cent of the latter showing a positive ^{125}I-fibrinogen test in at least one leg. Separate analysis shows that the blood changes are more severe in the major operation group (Fig. 1.3). The failure of the thrombosis group to show comparable differences can be accounted for if many patients with similar blood changes fail to develop thrombosis. The lack of any direct causal association between the changes and the incidence of thrombosis is further strengthened if time relationships are considered. Eighty per cent

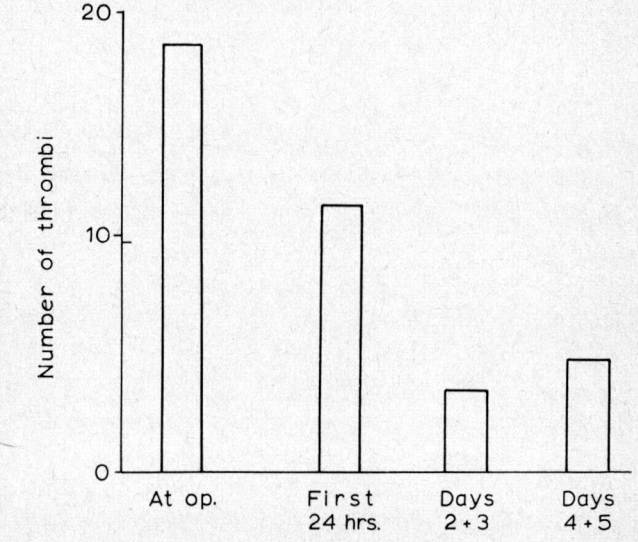

FIG. 1.4. The time thrombi were first detected in 27 patients (39 limbs) by the ^{125}I-fibrinogen test.

of the thrombi in this series were detected during the first 24 hours after operation (Fig. 1.4). Some blood changes were already apparent but the maximum increases in fibrinogen, lysis time, and FDP were from the second to the sixth day. Platelet adhesiveness was maximal from the third to the sixth day in the patients not receiving dextran, and platelet count highest on the sixth day.

COMMENT

It appears, therefore, that the changes observed in the plasma fibrinogen, blood lysis time, serum FDP, platelet count, and platelet adhesiveness, taken alone or together, fail to discriminate between those patients who have a thrombus and those who do not. These changes should be regarded as a sequel to surgical operation, more obvious in major than in minor operations, and not as indicative of venous thromboembolism. The known high incidence of thrombosis in the post-operative period makes it likely that they are associated with a 'hypercoagulable state' but they are more likely to represent one of its results rather than to be its cause. Since the blood changes differ in time from the period of maximum thrombus formation, their presence cannot be used to define the duration of the hypercoagulable state.

There is thus no evidence from these results to contradict the hypothesis that a change in the direction of hypercoagulability is a common, if not universal, event following the 'stress' of surgery. Thrombosis of a vein is an additional feature which may not occur unless other factors, perhaps harmless in themselves, are superimposed. The most important of such factors is probably blood flow in the veins. The dangers of stasis during a period of hypercoagulability have for long been emphasised by Wessler (1962). It is to be hoped that the promise of adequate prophylaxis for this crippling and sometimes fatal disorder may soon be achieved, perhaps by a combination of attempts to reduce blood clotting and improve blood flow.

REFERENCES

AMUNDSEN, M. A. et al. (1963) Ann. Int. Med., **58,** 608.
ATKINS, P. and HAWKINS, L. A. (1969) Surg. Gyne. Obst., **128,** 818.
BARKHAN, P. (1969) Brit. J. Haem., **17,** 221.
BENNETT, P. N. (1967) J. Clin. Path., **20,** 708.
BERGENTZ, S. E. and NILSSON, I. M. (1961) Acta Chir. Scand., **122,** 21.
BOROWIECKI, B. and SHARP, A. A. (1969) J. Trauma, **9,** 522.
BRECHER, G. and CRONKITE, E. P. (1950) J. App. Physiol., **3,** 365.
CASH, J. D. et al. (1969) Brit. med. J., **2,** 576.
DAVIDSON, E. and TOMLIN, S. (1963) J. Clin. Path., **16,** 112.
DAVIES, J. W. L. et al. (1970) Injury, **1,** 178.
EGEBERG, O. (1962) Acta Med. Scand., **171,** 679.
FEARNLEY, G. R. et al. (1957) Clin. Science, **16,** 645.
FLANC, C. et al. (1969) Lancet, **1,** 477.
FLUTE, P. T. (1965) Ann. Roy. Coll. Surg. Engl., **36,** 225.
FLUTE, P. T. (1970) J. Clin. Path., **23,** Suppl. (Royal Coll. Path.), **4,** 102.
GODAL, H. C. (1962) Acta Med. Scand., **171,** 687.
GORMSEN, J. and HAXHOLDT, B. F. (1960) Acta Chir. Scand., **120,** 121.
HAM, J. M. and SLACK, W. W. (1967) Brit. J. Surg., **54,** 385.
HARDAWAY, R. M. (1967) Amer. J. Cardiol., **20,** 161.
HARDAWAY, R. M. (1970) J. Clin. Path., **23,** Suppl. (Roy. Coll. Path.), **4,** 110.
HELLEM, A. J. (1960) Scand. J. Clin. Lab. Invest., **12,** Suppl. 51.

HELLEM, A. J. (1968) *Series Haem.*, **1,** 99.
HEWSON, W. (1772, repr. 1846) In *The Works of William Hewson, FRS*, ed. Gulliver, G., p. 46. London: Sydenham Society.
HICKMAN, J. A. (1971) *Clin. Science*, **41,** 141.
INGRAM, G. I. C. (1961) *J. Clin. Path.*, **14,** 356.
INNES, D. and SEVITT, S. (1964) *J. Clin. Path.*, **17,** 1.
KAKKAR, V. V. et al. (1970a) *Lancet*, **1,** 540.
KAKKAR, V. V. et al. (1970b) *Amer. J. Surg.*, **120,** 529.
KOWALSKI, E. (1968) *Sem. Haematology*, **5,** 45.
LEANDOER, L. (1968) *Acta Chir. Scand. Suppl.* 390.
LIM, R. C. Jr. et al. (1969) *Acta Chir. Scand.*, **135,** 363.
LIPINSKI, B. and WOROWSKI, K. (1968) *Thromb. Diath. Haem. (Stuttgart)*, **20,** 44.
MCKAY, D. G. (1969) *J. Trauma*, **9,** 646.
MERSKEY, C. et al. (1966) *Blood*, **28,** 1.
MERSKEY, C. et al. (1969) *Proc. Soc. Exp. Biol. Med.*, **131,** 871.
OLSSON, P. (1963) *Acta Chir. Scand.*, **126,** 24.
OLSSON, P. et al. (1964) *Acta Chir. Scand.*, **127,** 578.
PENICK, G. D. et al. (1965) *Fed. Proc.*, **24,** 835.
PENICK, G. D. (1966) *Thromb. Diath. Haem. (Stuttgart)*, Suppl. **21,** 543.
PHILLIPS, L. L. et al. (1963) *Ann. Surg.*, **157,** 317.
PISON, J. et al. (1965) *J. Amer. Med. Assoc.*, **191,** 1026.
PRENTICE, C. R. M. et al. (1969) *J. Clin. Path.*, **22,** 367.
RUCKLEY, C. V. et al. (1970) *Brit. med. J.*, **4,** 395.
SHARNOFF, J. G. et al. (1960) *Surg. Gyne. Obst.*, **111,** 469.
WESSLER, S. (1962) *Amer. J. Med.*, **33,** 648.
WESSLER, S. et al. (1967) *Thromb. Diath. Haem. (Stuttgart)*, **18,** 12.
WESSLER, S. and YIN, E. T. (1968) *Prog. Haematology*, **6,** 201.
WRIGHT, H. P. (1942) *J. Path. Bact.*, **54,** 461.
YGGE, J. (1970) *Amer. J. Surg.*, **119,** 225.
YIN, E. T. et al. (1971) *J. Biol. Chem.*, **246,** 3694.

2 The Issue of Hypercoagulability
S. Wessler*

In 1965 Freiman, Suyemoto and I in the New England Journal of Medicine, described the results of our dissection studies of the pulmonary arteries in 61 consecutive autopsied patients in a University General Hospital. Recent and organised thrombi ranging from massive emboli occluding the pulmonary arteries to minute, adherent, and barely visible fragments were found in 64 per cent of the cases studied. Since there is strong experimental evidence from our laboratory (Freiman et al., 1961) that the embolic traces observed at autopsy may represent only a small portion of the thrombotic material reaching the lung during life, this reported incidence may, in fact, be low.

In 1971 Nicolaides, Kakkar and their associates in the British Medical Journal demonstrated, by venous limbs scans, a 68 per cent incidence of deep leg vein thrombosis among severely ill patients admitted to a coronary intensive care unit and followed for 10 days. Recognising the restrictions of the technique and the limited number of days of study, this incidence, too, may well be low.

In further support of the ubiquity of venous thromboembolism are data demonstrating that the annual death rates from pulmonary embolism had risen between 1941 and 1961 (that is, after World War II and before the advent of antiovulatory agents) and again climbed during the past decade among men as well as women (Morell et al., 1963; Sherry et al., 1969).

Most of us have not been surprised by this further unmasking of the clinical segment of the thromboembolic iceberg. In what manner, however, should we respond to this cumulative evidence of the thromboembolic epidemic—beyond confirming what discerning pathologists have already told us?

In the first place, for the death rate findings to be interpretable, we must turn to the pathophysiologists.

*Supported in part by Research Grant HE 11470 from the National Heart and Lung Institute, National Institutes of Health; the American Heart Association, the Stella H. Shoenberg Research Fund, and the Sig and Clara Wolfort Research Fund.

What, in fact, *are* the criteria for deciding that pulmonary emboli are:
1. the cause of death
2. contributory to death, or
3. incidental to death?

Most pathologists smile when asked this question, but they rarely speak!

What further insights can we gain into the extent of the thromboembolic problem by examining the therapeutic effects of the classical anticoagulant drugs?

A number of conditions for which heparin and the coumarin compounds have been recommended as effective antithrombotic agents are listed in Table 2.1

TABLE 2.1

* Acute myocardial infarction	**Phlebitis
* Old myocardial infarction	**Pulmonary embolus
Coronary failure	Pulmonary thrombus
Angina pectoris	Pulmonary hypertension
Stroke complete	**Hip fracture
Stroke in progress	Post-partum
* Transient ischaemic attacks	Pelvic surgery
**Cerebral embolus	Atrial fibrillation reversion
**Acute peripheral arterial occlusion	* Valve prosthesis
Intermittent claudication	**DIC

** = marked benefit from anticoagulation
* = slight benefit from anticoagulation

These include cardiac, cerebral and peripheral arterial lesions, and peripheral venous and pulmonary arterial lesions as well as several categories of patients who are at special risk from thromboembolism. Those marked with a double asterisk represent conditions in which the data reflect an unequivocal benefit from anticoagulant therapy, although in some of the situations modifying clauses are necessary, such as 'hip fractures' which refers to individuals over the age of 45 who will remain bedridden for more than a few days.

Those marked with a single asterisk represent conditions in which the gain from anticoagulants is slight: in the case of acute and old myocardial infarction probably due to the decrease in pulmonary or systemic emboli. Moreover, there is a reasonable doubt as to the value of anticoagulants beyond 6 months following recovery from acute myocardial infarction. In the remaining disease states the value of anticoagulants is either indeterminate or nil.

It is apparent from this formulation that heparin and the coumarin drugs originally were overrated in terms of their antithrombotic capabilities. They are moderately effective on the venous side of the circulation and less so on the arterial side particularly in organs, such as the heart and brain, that have physiologically end-arterial circulations. Thus, successful therapy, directed toward arterial thromboemboli, is achieved largely in the extremities where, because of the rich, pre-formed interarterial circulation, extensive intravascular coagulation is necessary to produce arterial insufficiency. Therapy with heparin or coumarin compounds is also effective in the microcirculation in preventing or retarding disseminated intravascular coagulation.

From the results of conventional anticoagulant therapy alone, distinctions between arterial and venous thrombi present themselves, and it is apparent from a therapeutic view that disseminated intravascular coagulation has more in common with venous than with arterial lesions.

What must also be made clear is that, although venous thromboembolism is extremely common, the mortality from this condition is not great. All the new diagnostic tools: pulmonary angiography, lung scanning, pulmonary haemodynamics, the mechanics of respiration, phlebography and venous leg scans document a high frequency, but not a high mortality.

The urgency of the physician's concern with acute peripheral venous thrombosis, however, lies in the intimate but unpredictable association between thrombi in peripheral veins and the fatal embolization of these thrombi to the pulmonary arteries. In this context, both venous thrombosis and pulmonary embolism are best viewed as related, common conditions involving intravascular coagulation, in which the clinical diagnosis is often difficult, the prognosis usually good, the tendency to recurrence great, and the mortality, though relatively infrequent, quite unpredictable. If this be true, then it follows that many patients will have to be subjected unnecessarily to prophylactic therapy to protect the few from thromboembolic catastrophes and that the risks of therapy must be less than that of the disease.

It is this concern over not recognising the disease, coupled with the need to overtreat—particularly when the therapy itself represents some hazard—that has attracted great interest recently in defining populations at a high enough risk so that all in the group could be subjected to prophylactic therapy regardless of whether a diagnosis of venous thrombosis was or was not made in any particular patient in the group.

Certain risk factors, among others, have been fairly well identified: age, immobilization and bed rest, prior venous thromboembolism or arterial insufficiency, congestive heart failure, shock, oestrogens, gram negative sepsis, trauma including injury, surgery, and parturition, cancer and blood groups.

But what are the mechanisms whereby these risk factors may operate?

Venous thrombi do not occur indiscriminately throughout the body. They form in multiple, independent, bilateral sites of origin within the deep venous tree of the lower limbs, initially at valve pockets and dilated saccules occurring at vein junctions—all areas of relatively retarded blood flow.

Phlebographic and post-mortem data have suggested that with advancing age, the soleal veins and arcades increase in number, diameter and tortuosity—representing perhaps one basis for the increased risk of thrombosis attributable to age, *per se*. When increased age is combined with immobilization or bed rest, the supine position and the associated lack of muscle contraction accentuate the large dilated venous arcades and blood in the soleal veins is further stagnated. Similarly, previous venous thrombi, through residual obstruction to venous return, favour stasis. Patients who have a decrease in arterial limb perfusion or an increase in venous blood volume suffer from a reduction in linear flow velocity in the deep veins. Such rheological changes also promote stasis. In short, any factor slowing blood flow puts that individual at increased risk from venous thromboembolism.

Oestrogens administered to eliminate the pregnant state (Salhanick *et al.*, 1969), to prevent post-partum lactation (Daniel *et al.*, 1967), or employed for the treatment of coronary artery disease (Stamler—personal communication), or for the alleviation of metastatic carcinoma of the prostate (The Veterans Administration Co-operative Urological Research Group, 1967) are associated with an increase in thromboembolism and death—these findings in the latter two conditions, at least, being dose related. Oestrogens induce, aside from fluid retention, increased venous dilatation and distensibility thereby contributing to stagnant flow. Whether they have a role via hypercoagulability is unknown.

Gram negative sepsis is often associated with endotoxaemia which can, of course, produce both the local and generalized Shwartzman reactions as well as shock. All these actions can involve intravascular coagulation as an integral component. Though the precise mechanism remains an enigma, endothelial injury as well as stasis and hypercoagulability have been suggested as being responsible for the observed thrombogenicity.

Certain malignancies, particularly pancreas and lung, may predispose to venous thromboembolism. As to mechanism we have some fancy; but very little fact. The evidence for hypercoagulability has been disappointing.

Among women on the pill who develop venous thromboembolism, there is a significant deficit of individuals of the Group O blood type (Jick *et al.*, 1969). This skew of the ABO blood groups among patients with phlebitis on the pill has been subsequently reported in other groups of patients with venous thromboembolic disease (Talbot *et al.*, 1970). Whether there is a genetic factor here related

TABLE 2.2

Risk factor	Flow	Mechanism Intima	Coagulation
Age	+		
Immobilization, bed rest	+		
Prior venous thromboembolism, arterial insufficiency	+		
Congestive heart failure, shock	+		
Oestrogen	+		?
Gram negative sepsis	?	?	?
Trauma		+	
Cancer			?
Blood group			?

to hypercoagulability cannot be answered; yet, in this regard, it is well to recall, in that rare inborn error of sulphur amino-acid metabolism, homocystinuria, that the common mode of death in affected children is thrombosis.

When these risk factors are reduced to three common denominators it is, perhaps, ironic to note, as seen in Table 2.2, that most factors operate via retarded flow, one major category operates by way of intimal injury; whereas none can be established to operate through hypercoagulability.

I say ironic because, although this cumulative association of stasis and thrombosis appears valid, data both in animals and in man indicate that retarded blood flow alone does *not* initiate intravascular coagulation. If this be true, some alteration of the circulating constituents of the blood must be present to trigger intravascular coagulation in areas of retarded blood flow devoid of intimal injury.

If clotting factors do have a role in either the initiation or propagation of thrombi, stasis facilitates the progress of intravascular coagulation by at least four mechanisms: first, by protecting such thrombogenic species from dispersion; second, by impeding their neutralization by circulating inhibitors; and third, by impairing their clearance by the liver. Finally, retarded blood flow favours intravascular coagulation by profoundly altering the physical and chemical properties of a column of blood so as to predispose to fibrin formation. In fact, the only mechanism opposing thrombosis in areas of retarded flow is fibrinolysis.

There are also difficulties with the intimal injury-platelet plug as the single prototype for all thrombosis. First, it has not been possible, in experimental animals, to induce the platelet thrombus to extend beyond the zones of endothelial injury. Second, while explaining how the white thrombus causes ischaemia, primarily in physiologically end-arterial circuits, such as the heart, brain, and kidney, where even complete vessel occlusion is not required, this model fails to account for the extensive growth of red cell-fibrin coagula in the major veins and peripheral arteries or for fibrin deposits in the microcirculation as a result of disseminated intravascular coagulation.

Venous thrombi, although perhaps requiring a platelet nidus for their origin, in many instances present essentially as red thrombi consisting principally of fibrin and erythrocytes with white blood cells and platelets randomly distributed. The morphology cannot be explained by an analogy to the haemostatic plug. With the scanning electron microscope the thrombus is readily seen to consist of biconcave erythrocytes bridged by spaghetti-like fibrin strands wherein one hardly sees a platelet or platelet debris.

Since neither trauma to the intima alone, nor retarded blood flow *per se* can account for the dramatic growth of such red thrombi, it is not unreasonable for investigators to seek some systemic alteration in the clotting mechanism that triggers the rapid evolution of the fibrin thrombus.

Alterations in *in vitro* coagulation assays found among patients with thrombosis have led some investigators to conclude that the observed changes represent evidence of 'systemic hypercoagulability' that is causally related to thrombus formation. Support for this concept has been collected from at least three types of observations: the absence or relative rarity of phlebitis among patients with congenital deficiencies in specific clotting factors; the prophylactic efficacy of anticoagulant drugs; and the observed plasma elevations of specific clotting factors in the immediate post-partum period.

Objections to the validity of these arguments can, however, be readily marshalled. Thus, the data on patients with congenital deficiencies are scanty and include few individuals in the older age groups. Moreover, thrombosis has been observed in patients with low levels of Factors I, V, VII, and XII.

In regard to anticoagulant therapy, the fact that interference with clotting reactions can prevent thrombosis does not establish *a priori* that the basis for this effect is related to the prevention of a state of systemic hypercoagulability. Pregnant women in the third trimester have coagulation factor elevations of the same order as that found in the immediate post-partum period, yet a smaller incidence of phlebitis is observed during pregnancy than following delivery. In addition, many patients develop phlebitis without any detectable change in their coagulation profile, whereas others show changes in clotting factors that appear to be consequent rather than causal to the thrombosis.

Although it might reasonably be argued that a several-fold increase in a circulating clotting factor would set the stage for a greater and more rapid explosion of enzyme coagulation kinetics, no data in man or in animals have provided evidence to support this hypothesis.

Several years ago experiments in our laboratory demonstrated, with highly purified preparations of clotting factors, that it is not the quantity *per se* but rather the species of a clotting factor that is responsible for the initiation of thrombosis (Wessler and Yin, 1968). Thus, infusions into fasted rabbits of nonactivated Factor X in amounts up to 630 units failed to induce stasis thrombi. In contrast, as little as 5 units of activated Factor X were fully thrombogenic. These data indicate that whereas an infusion of nonactivated Factor X equivalent to the injection into rabbits of more than one litre of bovine plasma was inert, the infusion of an amount of this activity that can be derived from 10 ml of bovine plasma was thrombogenic. These findings support the view that hypercoagulability can be defined as a state in which activated coagulation products or intermediates, normally absent from circulating blood, are formed intravascularly.

This definition implies that, somewhere along the coagulation cascade, a proteolytic event has taken place, i.e., the enzymatic clotting sequence has been activated. This definition of hypercoagulability will not recognise the 'at risk' or 'thrombosis prone' patient in whom identification is based on a prior overall statistical judgement before subjecting the patient to a procedure associated with intravascular coagulation. This definition will also not recognise the patient in whom intravascular coagulation has ceased and in whom all compensatory biochemical mechanisms have returned to normal. On the other hand this definition could encompass the patient whose clotting mechanism has been activated, but in whom insufficient fibrin may have been laid down to be recognised by dye or isotope.

As a clinician, I believe I would be in a more effective position to begin antithrombotic therapy early if I could determine by a plasma assay that my patient were hypercoagulable (that is: the cascade trigger had somehow been pulled) than by waiting to visualise directly or indirectly that a thrombus had already been deposited in a vein.

What is the value of knowing so early that a patient is hypercoagulable? After all, no one ever died because a 5 or 10 ml thrombus from a tibial vein migrated to the pulmonary arteries; and have not Barritt and Jordan (1960) shown that even after the development of a clinically recognisable pulmonary embolus, heparin and coumarin drugs can save lives. Although these rejoinders have validity, I, nevertheless, believe there may well be an advantage to being able to interrupt intravascular coagulation early on.

In experimental support of this thesis we have recently identified a potent, naturally-occurring inhibitor to activated Factor X in human plasma and serum (Yin and Wessler, 1969), a finding originally noted by Seegers (1962). Using a highly purified inhibitor to Factor X from rabbit plasma, we have demonstrated its enhancement by heparin (Yin and Wessler, 1970) and have shown that the biological activities, variously termed 'activated Factor X inhibitor', 'antithrombin III' and 'heparin cofactor activity', all belong to a single blood proteinase inhibitor with broad specificity, but whose primary physiological substrate is activated Factor X (Wessler and Yin, 1970; Yin *et al.*, 1970). With *in vitro* experiments we have recently demonstrated that 1 µg of activated Factor X inhibitor, by inhibiting 32 units of activated Factor X, can indirectly prevent the potential generation of 1600 NIH units of thrombin.

In addition, more heparin is required to bring about instantaneous blockade of the thrombin-fibrinogen reaction by the inhibitor, than is required to neutralize activated Factor X irreversibly. These data emphasise that the coagulation enzymatic sequence functions as a biochemical amplifier. Accordingly, it would be reasonable to expect that, if hypercoagulability were treated early, it would require, for example, less of an antithrombotic agent, than if therapy were instituted later.

In the search for evidence of hypercoagulability the trail has moved away from overall screening assays because they have not been helpful, from non-activated clotting factors because these species are not thrombogenic, and from activated clotting species because they do not linger unaltered in the circulation. The search for the 'holy-grail' has properly shifted to the recognition of increments in relatively stable reaction products of coagulation or to alterations in stable clotting factor inhibitors.

In this regard, the findings of Fletcher and his associates are of particular interest (Fletcher and Alkjaersig, 1969). They have developed a method to provide data on fibrinogen/fibrin complexes and their derivatives in plasma. Their original and provocative plasma chromatographic technique offers promise of reflecting thrombosis, and its further development will be watched with great interest.

In another potential assay the initial stages of normal fibrinogen catabolism in animals have been described by Sherman to proceed by two pathways: one by limited fibrinogenolysis and the other by limited fibrin formation (cryofibrinogen) (Sherman and Fletcher, 1969). It is possible that the balance between the fibrin and lytic pathways may prove helpful in studying both the pathogenesis of thrombosis and in identifying the hypercoagulable patient.

An alternative approach is to determine whether changes in inhibitor levels to specific activated clotting proteins may not reflect hypercoagulability. For many years antithrombin-III (progressive antithrombin) has been considered by numerous investigators to be the principal circulating inhibitor to thrombin. Antithrombin-III levels vary considerably among different age groups and there are differences between health and disease (Abildgaard, 1968; von Kaulla and von Kaulla, 1967). Congenital deficiencies of this inhibitor in a family have also been reported and in these instances the members of the family have been thrombophilic (Ekberg, 1965). It has also been observed that the antithrombin-III level is reduced in women on oral contraceptive agents (von Kaulla and von Kaulla, 1970; Peterson et al., 1970).

Our data strongly suggest, first, that the key function of activated Factor X inhibitor or antithrombin III as a natural anticoagulant is primarily concerned with the regulation of the haemostatic balance through neutralization of activated Factor X rather than of thrombin, and, second that the primary function of heparin is to facilitate the anticoagulant action of the inhibitor to activated Factor X, rather than its blocking the thrombin-fibrinogen reaction (Wessler and Yin, 1970; Yin et al., 1970). Several of these findings have recently been confirmed by other investigators (Biggs et al., 1970). Studies are now in progress to determine whether changes in the level of this inhibitor can, in fact, reflect hypercoagulability.

Just as the hypercoagulability story remains illusive, so does the answer to the initiation of intravascular coagulation remain shrouded in mystery. The elucidation of this latter issue may, however, shed light on the recognition of the hypercoagulable state.

It has been demonstrated, in many laboratories and over a long span of years, that the infusion into mammals of one or more activated clotting factors will induce intravascular coagulation. Thrombosis may also be initiated experimentally by substances that are not themselves activated clotting proteins, but that apparently have the capacity to initiate such protein activation. These include: tissue thromboplastin, trypsin, fatty acids, the diatomaceous earth, celite, ellagic acid and endotoxin.

Among these substances, interest in endotoxin as a potential trigger stems from the fact, already mentioned, that it not only produces thrombosis in man and in animals, but may enter the systemic circulation intermittently during shock.

Although considerable data are available describing the effects of endotoxin on platelets and clotting proteins, little information has been obtained regarding the molecular basis for these events.

A priori, endotoxin-induced coagulation must involve at least one proteolytic event—that is, the conversion of fibrinogen to fibrin. From this requirement one can speculate that the initial step in endotoxin-induced coagulation may involve the formation of an active complex capable of catalyzing the activation of a clotting protein. This would result in the activation of the remaining zymogens in the clotting sequence ending in the formation of a fibrin gel.

Recently, Müeller-Eberhard (1971) has demonstrated complex formation between endotoxin and a β-globulin component of normal serum that is capable of activating complement, which, like the coagulation sequence, involves a series of proteolytic events. These observations suggest a possible molecular basis for endotoxin-induced thrombosis and, by extension, a tool to recognise hypercoagulability.

In conclusion, I should like to urge that we not turn our backs on clinical observations. Thrombosis in sickle cell disease is common, but pulmonary embolism is rare; thrombosis in polycythemia vera is frequent, yet pulmonary embolism is almost unheard of; venous thrombosis in uncomplicated thyrotoxicosis is yet to be reported. These statements still belong to the era of anecdotal medicine. The relation between venous thromboembolism and blood groups has, however, received statistical support. There are messages here that have still to be decoded.

These observations together with the advances in electron microscopy, enzymology, rheology and isotopes still leave the problem of hypercoagulability in the era of the xerox machine; it is to be hoped, with all the burgeoning new interdisciplinary knowledge, that the hypercoagulability issue will soon enter the age of the computer.

REFERENCES

ABILDGAARD, U. (1968) *Scand. J. Clin. Lab. Invest.*, **21**, 89.
BARRITT, D. W. and JORDAN, S. C. (1960) *Lancet*, **1**, 1309.
BIGGS, R. et al. (1970) *Brit. J. Haemat.*, **19**, 283.
DANIEL, D. G. et al. (1967) *Lancet*, **2**, 287.
EKBERG, O. (1965), *Thromb. Diath. Haemorrh.*, **13**, 516.
FLETCHER, A. P. and ALKJAERSIG, N. (1969) *J. Lab. Clin. Med.*, **74**, 873.
FREIMAN, D. G. et al. (1961) *Am. J. Path.*, **39**, 95.
FREIMAN, D. G. et al. (1965) *New Eng. J. Med.*, **272**, 1278.
JICK, H. et al. (1969) *Lancet*, **1**, 539.
VON KAULLA, E. and VON KAULLA, K. N. (1967) *Am. J. Clin. Path.*, **48**, 69.
VON KAULLA, E. and VON KAULLA, K. M. (1970) *Lancet*, **1**, 36.
MORRELL, M. T. et al. (1963) *Brit. Med. J.*, **2**, 830.
MÜLLER-EBERHARD, H. J. (1971) *Fed. Proc.*, **30**, 184.
NICOLAIDES, A. N. et al. (1971) *Brit. med. J.*, **1**, 432.
PETERSON, R. et al. (1970) *Am. J. Clin. Path.*, **53**, 468.
SALHANICK, H. A. et al. (ed.) (1969) *Metabolic Effects of Gonadal Hormones and Contraceptive Steriods.* New York: Plenum Press.
SEEGERS, W. H. and MARCINIAK, E. (1962) *Nature*, **193**, 1188.
SHERMAN, L. A. and FLETCHER, A. P. (1969) *J. Lab. Clin. Med.*, **73**, 574.
SHERRY, S. et al. (ed.) (1969) *Thrombosis.* Washington, D.C.: National Academy of Sciences.
STAMLER, J. Personal communication.
TALBOT, S. et al. (1970) *Lancet*, **1**, 1257.
The Veterans Administration Co-operative Urological Research Group (1967) *Surg. Gynec. Obst.*, **124**, 1011.
WESSLER, S. and YIN, E. T. (1968) *J. Lab. Clin. Med.* **72**, 256.
WESSLER, S. and YIN, E. T. (1970) *Circulation*, **42**, suppl. III, 48.
YIN, E. T. and WESSLER, S. (1969) *Thromb. Diath. Haemorrh.*, **21**, 398.
YIN, E. T. et al. (1970) *Blood*, **36**, 835.
YIN, E. T. and WESSLER, S. (1970) *Biochem. Biophys. Acta.*, **201**, 387.

3 Fibrinogen—Fibrin Degradation Products and Venous Thromboembolism

A. P. Fletcher*, N. Alkjaersig* and J. O'Brien

The urgent need for the development of blood assay methods capable of detecting the presence of *in vivo* thrombosis and/or blood hypercoagulability has long been obvious to both clinicians and investigators in the thromboembolic field. However, for reasons that are now well-understood, principally the rapid *in vivo* clearance of activated coagulation factors, the even more rapid *in vivo* inhibition of such factors and the indirect nature of information derived from assay of unactivated coagulation factors, blood coagulation assays, dependent on blood coagulation reactant quantification, have yielded only meagre dividend.

However, *in vivo* enzymatic reactions may be detected either by study of the reactants themselves or by quantification of specific reaction end-products. A logical approach to this problem, but one hitherto neglected because of daunting technical difficulties, would require the identification and quantification of specific reaction end-products, all derivatives of fibrinogen and/or fibrin, characteristic of *in vivo* thrombosis, blood hypercoagulability, intravascular coagulation or fibrinolysis.

Table 3.1 presents, in simplistic fashion, the diagnostic possibilities inherent in the reaction end-product approach.

Four situations may be envisaged—first, the case of the normal subject in whom plasma fibrinogen will essentially exist as a single molecular species of 330,000 molecular weight. Second, the patient with thrombosis in whom fibrin proteolysis products will circulate in plasma, because of the actions of the plasma fibrinolytic enzyme system on the thrombus. These proteolysis products complex both with themselves and/or fibrinogen, forming fibrinogen-fibrin proteolysis complexes of from 400,000 to 1 million molecular weight,

*Supported by USPHS HE–03745, NIH 69–2263, FDA 70–55, and NICHHD 71–6027.

but characteristically, with a mean molecular weight of around 450,000. Third, is the largely theoretical situation where true blood hypercoagulability exists in the absence of thrombosis—in this instance, fibrinogen-fibrin monomer dimers exhibiting a molecular weight of 660,000 will be found. Finally, as we showed some years ago (Fisher *et al.*, 1967), increased overall activity of the plasma fibrinolytic enzyme system—an enzyme system activated by thrombosis or intravascular coagulation—will be characterized by the presence of increased concentrations of fibrinogen first derivative (Fletcher *et al.*, 1966) in plasma—this derivative has a molecular weight of 267,000, rather than the 330,000 of fibrinogen.

TABLE 3.1

BIOCHEMICAL MARKERS FOR BLOOD HYPERCOAGULABILITY AND THROMBOSIS

Molecular weights of fibrinogen, derivatives and complexes characteristic of blood hypercoagulable and thrombotic states.

Patient state	Markers in plasma
Normal	Plasma fibrinogen is single molecular species of 330,000 M.W.
Thrombosis	Large molecular weight fibrinogen—fibrin proteolysis complexes (400,000–1 million M.W.).
Hypercoagulability	Large molecular weight fibrinogen—fibrin monomer complexes present, 660,000 M.W.
Fibrinolysis	Fibrinogen derivatives (267,000 M.W. or smaller).

Thus, large molecular weight fibrinogen complexes will be present in plasma during active thrombotic states, while during resolution, fibrinogen first derivative, of smaller molecular weight than fibrinogen itself, will be present.

Gel exclusion chromatography separates proteins on a molecular weight basis. Consequently, if plasma is gel chromatographed on precisely-calibrated columns of Biogel 5M and the effluent fractions are specifically assayed for fibrinogen, a plot of effluent fibrinogen concentration against effluent volume yields a plasma fibrinogen molecular weight distribution pattern (Fletcher *et al.*, 1970; Fletcher and Alkjaersig—in press). We use two specific fibrinogen assays for this purpose, a thrombin clottable method and an immunologic method; there is excellent concordance between these two assay methods.

The top of Fig. 3.1 shows the situation in the normal subject. Plasma fibrinogen is eluted as a symmetrical Gaussian-type curve, peaking at the column calibration point (the dotted line shown in all subsequent figures). This is an elution pattern characteristic of a single molecular weight species.

The presence of high molecular weight fibrinogen complexes shifts the elution pattern to the left (middle of Fig. 3.1) while the

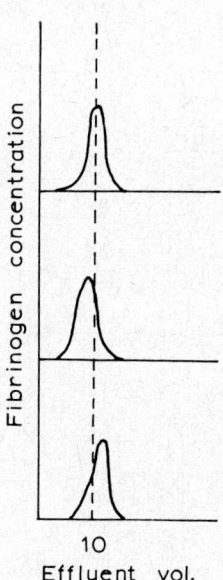

PLASMA FIBRINOGEN GEL ELUTION PATTERNS

NORMAL
  Gaussian Curve, single molecular species.

HYPERCOAGULABILITY/THROMBOSIS
  Large molecular weight complexes
  Pattern shift to left.

FIBRINOGENOLYSIS
  Derivatives smaller than fibrinogen
  Pattern shift to right
  Mixed patterns also occur

FIG. 3.1. Illustrative plasma fibrinogen chromatograms. Patient plasma is gel filtered on precisely-calibrated columns of Biogel 5M. Serial discrete effluent fractions are analysed for fibrinogen. The fibrinogen concentration (ordinate) is plotted against effluent volume (abscissa), yielding a plasma fibrinogen molecular weight distribution pattern.

presence of fibrinogen first derivative shifts the pattern to the right (bottom section of Fig. 3.1). Mixed patterns occur with great frequency.

Fig. 3.2 (from an *in vitro* study) displays three fibrinogen molecular weight distribution patterns from the same normal plasma; first, untreated (the solid circles), second, treated with urokinase prior to gel filtration (dotted line with open triangles) and lastly, the same normal plasma to which 1 mg/ml early fibrin proteolysis products had been added, prior to gel filtration—the last situation simulates the conditions in *in vivo* thrombosis.

The normal plasma shows a smooth symmetrical fibrinogen distribution pattern characteristic of a single molecular species and

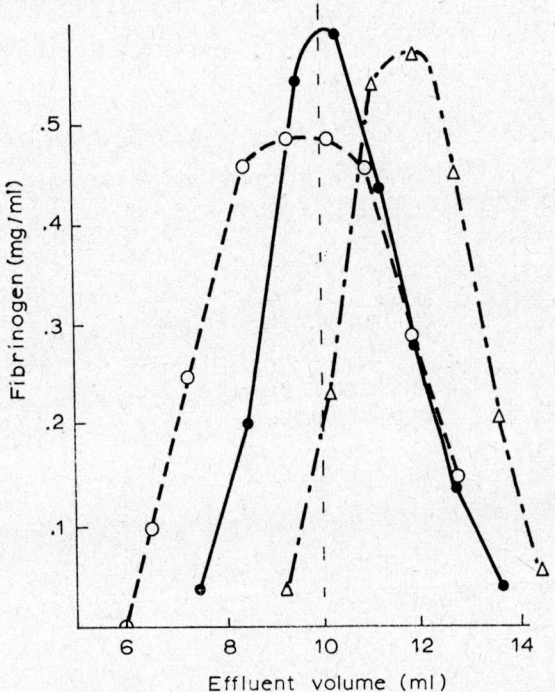

FIG. 3.2. Chromatograms of the same plasma, which, prior to chromatography, were either untreated, treated with urokinase, or treated with lysed fibrin, 1 mg/ml. The plasma treated with fibrin proteolysis products shows a broad pattern with a shift to the left, while the chromatogram from the plasma treated with urokinase is shifted to the right.

centred at the column calibration line. Plasma treated with small amounts of urokinase (open triangles) contains mainly fibrinogen first derivative of 267,000 molecular weight, rather than fibrinogen of 330,000 molecular weight and the whole distribution is shifted to the right.

In contrast (open circles, interrupted line) the addition of 1 mg/ml fibrin proteolysis products to normal plasma, results in the formation of high molecular weight fibrinogen-fibrin proteolysis complexes. Thus, the fibrinogen elution peak is both greatly broadened and shifted markedly to the left.

The plasma fibrinogen chromatogram is grossly altered in the presence of even the most minor thrombotic episode and, consequently, the chromatogram may either be interpreted visually by

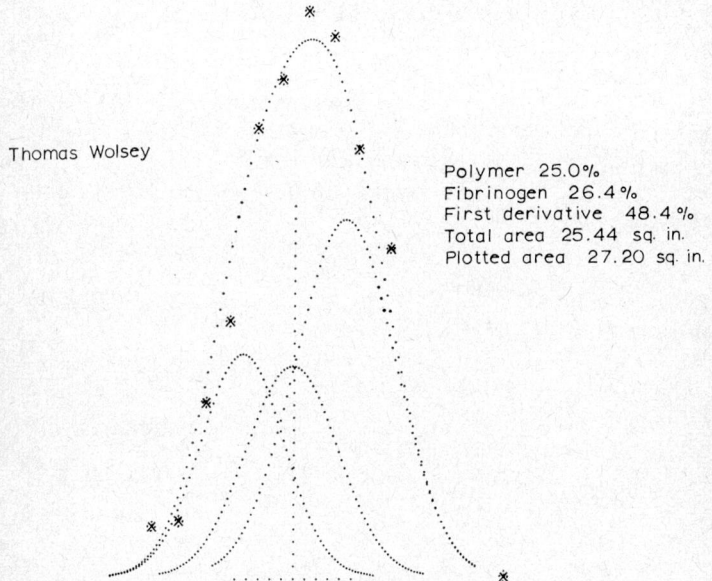

FIG. 3.3. A computer print-out and analysis of a chromatogram from a patient with post-operative thrombophlebitis. The asterisks show the original data points entered. The three overlapping lower curves, from left to right, represent analyses for polymer, fibrinogen and fibrinogen first derivative (analyses at experimentally-determined effluent volumes and using chromatographic plate theory). The curve close to the asterisks is the sum of the three lower curves.

the experienced investigator or by means of computer analysis. Obviously, the computer analysis possesses the advantage of providing wholly-objective interpretation and quantitative data. Fig. 3.3 shows such a computer analytical plot, the asterisks designating the original data points entered. The computer calculates and plots the best fitting curve for the data points and then, given three experimentally-determined effluent peak volumes—those for polymer, fibrinogen and fibrinogen first derivative—solves the problem of best Gaussian fit for these three components using Gaussian parameters, predicated on chromatographic plate theory—the three overlapping curves at the bottom of the figure. Print-out (right-hand bottom section of the figure) gives percentage individual component composition.

This analysis and print-out of chromatographic findings on plasma from a patient with thrombophlebitis shows that large molecular weight complexes, referred to as polymer, constitute 25 per cent of the whole, normal fibrinogen 26 per cent and fibrinogen first derivative 49 per cent. These findings are typical of a thrombotic lesion during resolution.

During 1966, Dr. Fedor Bachmann investigated a heat-stroke epidemic at St. Louis City Hospital; of 200 patients studied, 25 died with late thromboembolic complications. Using earlier versions of our present methods (Fletcher, 1967), we demonstrated in four patients succumbing to wholly-unexpected catastrophic pulmonary embolism that several days prior to death, high concentrations of large molecular weight fibrinogen complexes appeared and persisted in the plasma. These were highly encouraging findings for, clearly, we were detecting thrombosis in its early, clinically-silent, and treatable phase.

The pioneering work by Kakkar, Flanc, Browse, Flute and others from England on the detection of post-operative thrombophlebitis by isotopic means provided a potentially highly-suitable clinical model for the rigorous testing of our hypothesis that clinically-silent thrombosis was detectable by blood assay methods. Fortunately, this well-validated method for detecting post-operative thrombophlebitis came into large-scale use through Dr. John O'Brien's request to the British Medical Research Council for support of studies on drug prophylactic assessment in post-operative thromboembolism.

Table 3.2 outlines the collaborative study arranged between Dr. John O'Brien and ourselves. The clinical and isotopic studies were performed in Portsmouth and frozen plasma samples were shipped to St. Louis by air. Our laboratory studies were performed and interpreted without knowledge as to whether the patient developed thrombosis. However, the plasma fibrinogen chromatographic results were so strikingly altered in the presence of thrombosis that interpretive difficulties were minimal.

Fig. 3.4 depicts characteristic findings in a patient developing thrombophlebitis on post-operative day 1.

The pre-operative chromatogram on the left was normal and the isotopic leg scan was also normal. The disturbance of the chromatogram to the left on day 1 is obvious and this occurred concomi-

TABLE 3.2
DETECTION OF POST-OPERATIVE THROMBOPHLEBITIS
Schema of the co-operative study arranged between the Portsmouth and St. Louis laboratories.

1. Post-operatively .... ^{125}I labelled fibrinogen administered
2. Post-operatively .... Daily isotopic leg scanning
3. Thrombophlebitis diagnosed by detection of local isotope accumulation
4. Frozen plasma samples shipped to St. Louis

tantly with positivity of the leg scan. By post-operative day 4, the left limb of the chromatogram was clearly approaching normality and the right chromatographic limb shows the presence of excess fibrinogen first derivative. At this time, the isotopic leg scan was still abnormal, but the excess counts had fallen notably, indicating thrombus resolution, and the chromatographic pattern is also one of a resolving thrombus.

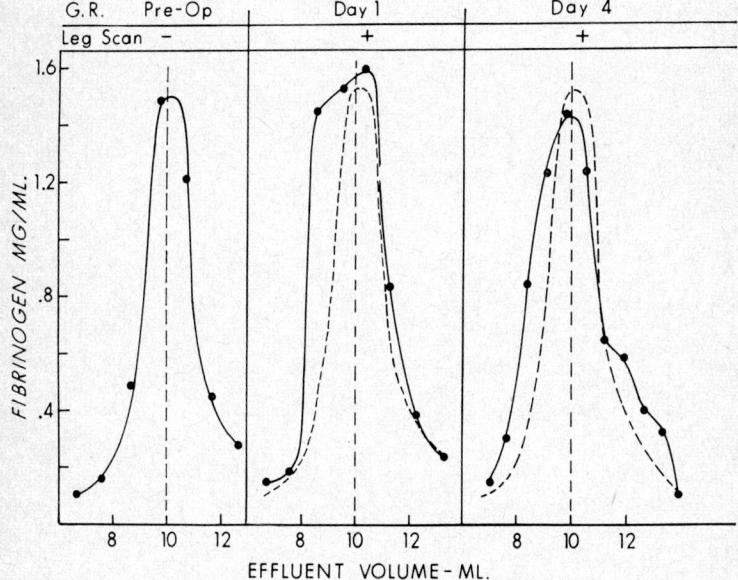

FIG. 3.4. Serial chromatographic and isotopic studies in a patient developing post-operative thrombophlebitis on day 1. Solid lines are actual chromatographic findings, the interrupted line in panels 2 and 3 is the pre-operative chromatogram examination findings shown for comparison purposes. See text for interpretation.

Fig. 3.5 shows isotopic data over a leg thrombus (top of figure) and computer analytical plots of our chromatographic data in the bottom section of the figure—these latter data are plotted as individual percentages for polymer, fibrinogen and fibrinogen first derivative.

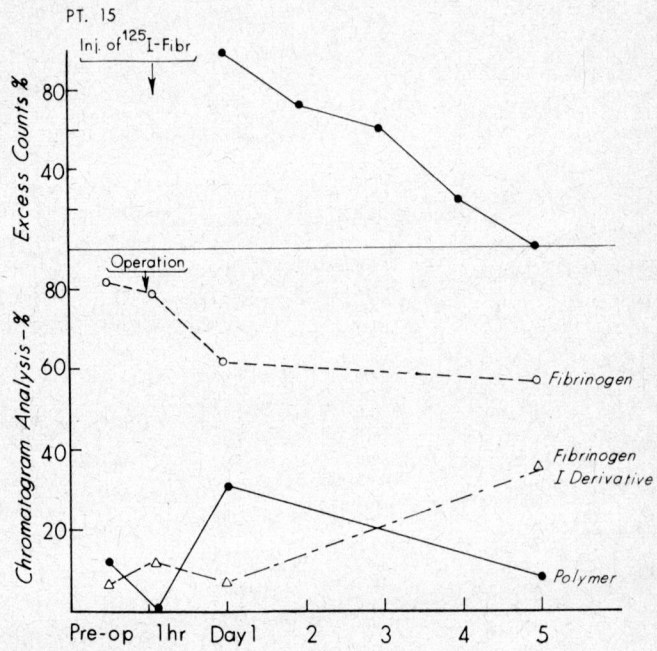

FIG. 3.5. Isotopic and computer chromatographic print-out data in a patient developing post-operative thrombosis on day 1. Note above, on day 1, the development of an isotopic 'hot' spot in the leg scan and below, the concomitant rise of polymer concentration to 35 per cent. On day 5, when the isotopic 'hot' spot had disappeared, polymer concentrations had fallen to the normal range, but fibrinogen first derivative concentration had risen sharply; the biochemical findings characteristic of a resolving thrombus.

A thrombus developed in this patient on post-operative day 1. Note the sudden appearance of excess counts over this leg area and the subsequent fall of counts over this site, indicative of complete thrombus resolution by day 5.

The initial chromatographic data on day 1 are diagnostic of thrombosis, showing a rapid rise of polymer to 25 per cent and a concomitant fall in uncomplexed fibrinogen. By day 5, when the thrombus was no longer detectable by isotopic means, polymer levels had fallen to within normal limits, but fibrinogen first derivative had risen to 38 per cent—the picture of a resolving thrombus.

Fig. 3.6 constructed on similar lines to Fig. 3.5, displays two additional study features. First, there is minor discrepancy between the radioactive scan data above and the chromatographic data

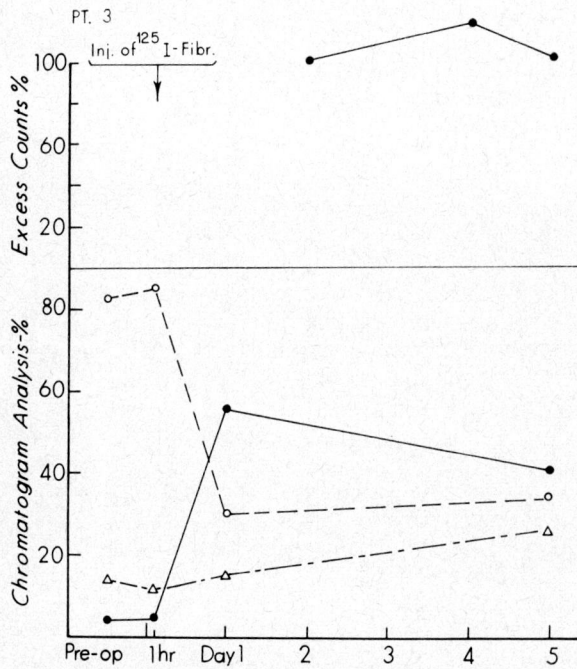

Fig. 3.6. Similar in construction to Fig. 3.5. Note that the diagnosis of thrombosis was made on day 1 by chromatography, but on day 2, by isotopic scanning. Note also that the isotopic scan data showed no change from day 1 to day 5; i.e., the clot did not resolve. Consequently, the lower figure section, polymer concentration remained grossly elevated at day 5.

below. We made a confident diagnosis of thrombosis from the chromatographic data on day 1—the rise of polymer to 55 per cent of the total—whereas radioactive findings did not show positivity until day 3. Also, the radioactive scan data demonstrate that the thrombus persisted during the observation period. Note that polymer levels also remained high during this same period, though the rise in fibrinogen first derivative shown on day 5 suggests that thrombolysis probably occurred shortly thereafter.

Overall, a highly satisfactory correlation was demonstrated to exist between the ^{125}I scan data and the plasma chromatographic results in the post-operative patient.

In 72 patients (left-hand section of Table 3.3), there was a complete agreement between the two methods, 31 patients being demonstrated to pass through the post-operative period without development of thrombophlebitis and 41 patients developing isotopic evidence of thrombophlebitis, together with appropriate plasma chromatographic changes. The right-hand section of Table 3.3 shows that major or minor discrepancies were recorded in 29 patients; in 22 of these, plasma chromatographic findings, diagnostic of thrombosis, were detected in the absence of confirmatory isotopic findings.

TABLE 3.3

IN VIVO ISOTOPIC SCAN FINDINGS *VERSUS* IN VITRO ASSAY

Correlation between *in vivo* isotopic scan findings and the plasma fibrinogen chromatographic data. See text for details.

Correlated (72 *pts*)		*Discrepant* (29 *pts*)	
Normal by both assays	*Abnormal by both assays*	*Normal* in vivo *Abnormal* in vitro	*Abnormal* in vivo *Normal* in vitro
31	41	22 (15 abnormal before Injection of ^{125}I)	7

However, this was a very high risk patient group, many with carcinoma of the lung and in 15 of the patients, evidence of thrombosis was detected by our plasma chromatographic method prior to the injection of the isotope. Since the chromatographic method detects thrombosis anywhere in the body, while the isotopic method is restricted to diagnosis of lower-limb thrombophlebitis, it is to be expected, especially in this clinical context, that thrombosis will be diagnosed substantially more frequently by plasma chromatographic methodology, rather than by local isotopic leg scanning.

Breakdown of the group of 7 patients in whom positive evidence of thrombophlebitis was obtained in the absence of wholly-concordant chromatographic data showed discrepancies to be minor.

This collaborative study demonstrates that the plasma fibrinogen chromatographic method is one of extraordinary sensitivity and accuracy for detecting *in vivo* thrombotic activity, together with its resolution. Thus, many problems, previously studied by epidemiological and other indirect means, becomes accessible to direct investigative study in small patient groups. I shall conclude by brief reference to studies on women receiving oral contraceptive medication—a most pressing problem.

Fig. 3.7 shows serial chromatographic studies on a 26 year-old woman receiving oral contraceptive medication for one year and admitted with a tentative diagnosis of pulmonary embolism. This diagnosis was not confirmed by lung scan, but the chromatographic

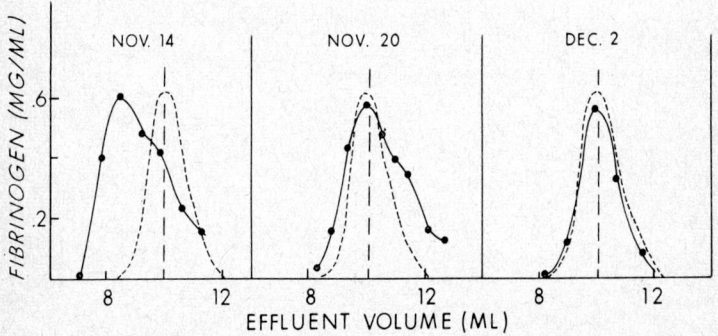

FIG. 3.7. Serial plasma fibrinogen chromatographic findings in a 26 year-old female on oral contraceptive medication for one year and admitted to the hospital with a tentative diagnosis of pulmonary embolism. This diagnosis was not confirmed, but note (left hand panel of the figure) chromatographic findings typical of a thrombotic lesion (middle of the figure), those typical of thrombus resolution and, in the right-hand panel, a return to normal plasma fibrinogen chromatographic findings.

data indicated first, the presence of a thrombus (left-hand figure section), second, its resolution (middle of figure) and then later, return to normal chromatographic findings. Such transient alterations in plasma fibrinogen chromatographic findings, usually lasting from 2-6 weeks and indicative of a thrombotic episode with subsequent resolution, occur frequently in subjects receiving oral contraceptive medication and relatively rarely in normals.

Table 3.4 summarizes 553 observations on 380 patients, some followed serially.

The data show that whereas in women not receiving oral contraceptive agents (the control group), the incidence of transient chromatographic abnormality was under 5 per cent, in those receiving oral contraceptive agents for less than six months it was 14 per cent, rising to between 17–23 per cent in those on medication from between six months to more than 4 years. Thus, our findings indicate that women receiving oral contraceptive medication experience episodes, usually asymptomatic, of a thrombotic nature with a frequency approximately 5-fold greater than do those women not receiving such therapy.

This risk frequency is similar to that determined from epidemiological study and would suggest that the increased risk of experiencing clinically-overt thromboembolism while on oral contraceptive

TABLE 3.4

Shows the incidence of plasma fibrinogen chromatographic abnormality in untreated patients (control patients) and in those receiving oral contraceptive medication over varying time periods.

	Number		Abnormal		% of	
	Obs.	Pts.	Obs.	Pts.	Obs.	Pts.
Control patients	107	106	5	4	4·7	3·7
Trial series						
Pts. on med. less than 6 months	102	51	14	9	13·8	17·6
Referred series						
On med. less than 1 year	35	30	6	5	17·1	16·7
On med. 1 to 4 years	130	108	30	22	23·0	20·3
On med. more than 4 years	179	136	42	30	23·4	22·0

TOTAL 553 observations on 380 patients

agents relates to an increased occurrence of generally clinically-silent thrombotic lesions, rather than to pathophysiological changes favouring thrombus extension.

During the recent Medical Research Council drug prophylactic trial on post-operative venous thromboembolism, only 22 per cent of those diagnosed as having thrombophlebitis by isotopic means developed signs or symptoms diagnostic of this condition.

Similarly, the great majority of patients in our present oral contraceptive trial series developed 'clinically-silent' thrombotic lesions diagnosable only by plasma chromatographic findings. However, symptomatic breakdown demonstrated significant association of symptoms suggestive of thromboembolism with plasma fibrinogen chromatographic abnormality.

Sixty-eight patients of the 380 patients followed were symptomatic at the time of examination and Table 3.5 shows the symptomatic breakdown.

Symptoms 1-4 were classified as not suggestive of thromboembolism while those marked 5-7 were classified as suggestive of thromboembolism. In the group of 33 patients suffering from non-thromboembolic symptoms, there were abnormal chromatographic

TABLE 3.5

SYMPTOMS—LONG TERM ORAL CONTRACEPTIVE MEDICATION SERIES

Symptomatic breakdown in those patients listed in Table 3.4. The incidence of plasma fibrinogen chromatographic abnormality is significantly associated with symptoms suggestive of thromboembolic disease.

	Total	Abnormal Pattern	%
1. Gynaecological symptoms	12	2	16·5
2. Bruises and/or easy bruising	9	3	33
3. Headache	4	1	25
4. Unclassified complaints	8	0	
5. Varicose veins, symptomatic	4	2	50
6. Leg pains with or without swelling	22	10	45
7. Chest pain	9	6	67
TOTALS	68	24	

Symptoms not suggestive of thromboembolism
  Numbered 1-4: 33 patients, 6 abnormal patterns
Symptoms suggestive of thromboembolism
  Numbered 5-7: 35 patients, 18 abnormal patterns
  X^2 (with Yates correction) $= 6·82$ $p < 0·01$

findings in 6, while in the second group of 35 patients suffering from symptoms suggestive of thromboembolism, there were 18 exhibiting thrombotic hypercoagulable chromatographic patterns. X^2 with Yates correction 6·82 (p was less than 0·01) a highly significant association of symptoms suggestive of thromboembolism with abnormal plasma fibrinogen chromatographic findings.

These data suggest that we can now assess the relative *in vivo* thrombogenicity of various oral contraceptive regimens, using small patient groups (during the clinical investigative phase of drug testing) and prior to the marketing of the preparation.

This clearly is a considerable advance over the former method of exposing large populations to uncertain risk for considerable time periods for the purpose of collecting morbidity and mortality data.

COMMENT

First, the methods, in their present state of development, are intensely laborious and require an unusual degree of technical expertise and skill. Indeed, their use is presently and unfortunately, restricted to specialised skilled laboratories. However, recent technical developments, particularly our development of a computer programme for quantification, suggest that several, otherwise difficult, steps may now be automated by directly interfacing analytical instruments to the computer. Other types of simplification are also under development.

Second, I would emphasise that as useful as these methods are in the study of venous disease, their most important uses belong in two quite different fields: in the study of acute arterial syndromes—cerebral vascular disease (Fletcher and Alkjaersig, 1971), myocardial infarction, etc., and in the prescription and control of therapeutic agents acting on the coagulation and fibrinolytic enzyme systems, e.g. thrombolytic agents and anticoagulant agents.

Finally, as must now be obvious, it is clear that these methods are only highly specific with respect to the pathological process examined and the results must in all cases be interpreted within the relative clinical context. Nevertheless, despite this caveat, practical experience demonstrates that interpretative difficulties are relatively few.

REFERENCES

FISHER, S. et al. (1967) *J. Lab. Clin. Med.*, **70,** 903.
FLETCHER, A. et al. (1966) *J. Lab. Clin. Med.* **68,** 780.
FLETCHER, A. P. (1967) *Thromb. et Diath. Haemorrh. Suppl.* **26,** 343.
FLETCHER, A. et al. (1970) *Transactions of the Assoc. of Am. Physicians*, **83,** 159.
FLETCHER, A. and ALKJAERSIG, N. (1971) *Houston Symposium on Stroke*, in press.
FLETCHER, A. and ALKJAERSIG, N. (1971) *Thromb. et Diath. Haemorrh.*, Suppl. Immunological Mechanisms in Blood Coagulation, Thrombosis and Haemostasis, p. 389.

ory Tests for the
                    Venous
                    olism

The early clinical recognition of thrombotic disorders has been severely handicapped by a lack of reliable laboratory tests. Thrombosis is apt to be recognised only after vascular occlusion has caused tissue damage and compromised organ function. The haematologic detection of thrombotic or prethrombotic states has been thwarted by the efficiency with which procoagulants are inactivated or cleared from the circulation. Clotting factors in their inactive state are normally present in considerable excess and, therefore, determination of their levels in the blood has been of limited clinical value, except in the diagnosis of haemorrhagic disorders.

A more hopeful approach to the laboratory detection of thrombosis involves the measurement of certain fibrinogen derivatives which remain in the circulation. Fibrin monomers and fibrin degradation products represent two coagulation products whose presence in the blood specifically reflects the elaboration of thrombin. Thrombin itself is too rapidly inactivated to be detected. The enzymatic action of thrombin on fibrinogen results in the formation of fibrin monomer. This molecule is capable of polymerization resulting in fibrin formation. However, this final step is inhibited by the formation of soluble complexes composed of fibrin monomers and fibrinogen or fibrinogen degradation products. Polymerization is thereby prevented, representing perhaps the body's final anticlotting defence. When fibrin is lysed by plasmin, the resultant early fibrin degradation products are similarly capable of spontaneous polymerization which also is prevented by the formation of soluble complexes with fibrinogen and fibrinogen degradation products.

As shown schematically (Fig. 4.1), the presence of these complexes in the blood is specific evidence of thrombin elaboration and incipient or overt fibrin formation. In the presence of appropriate concentrations of protamine sulphate, these complexes are known to dissociate resulting in fibrin formation (Kopec et al., 1962). This nonenzymatic fibrin formation has been termed paracoagulation (Derechin et al., 1955). The serial dilution protamine sulphate or SDPS test takes advantage of the biological property of fibrin monomers and early fibrin degradation products to polymerize spontaneously when dissociated from their complexes. The test differs from other methods in that it utilises much smaller concentrations of protamine sulphate than previously employed and a

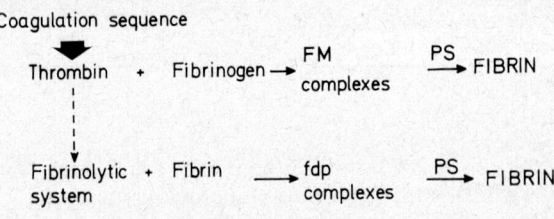

FIG. 4.1. Paracoagulation.

diluted plasma system which are essential for both specificity and sensitivity. The test is semiquantitative and both simpler and more sensitive than other published methods. Serial dilutions of protamine sulphate ranging from 1:5 to 1:40 are made with 0·05M Tris buffer at pH 6·5 and added to equal volumes of citrated platelet poor plasma to which one drop of aprotinin (Trasylol) has been added. The test is read after 30 minutes and again after 24 hours standing corked at room temperature. Both the use of the buffer and the increased time represent modifications of the SDPS test since its original publication (Niewiarowski and Gurewich, 1971).

TABLE 4.1

SDPS TEST RESULTS

SDPS test in the presence of fibrinogen, fibrinogen degradation products (FDP), fibrin degradation products (fdp) and fibrin monomers (FM).

mg % in plasma				SDPS
Fibrinogen	FDP	FM	fdp	
200–500	—	—	—	+
	400	—	—	—
		1·0	—	fs or g
			0·5	fs or g

The formation of a fibrin strand precipitate (represented by fs) or a gel (represented by g) is specific for the presence of fibrin monomers or early fibrin degradation products (Table 4.1).

Fibrinogen forms an amorphous, granular precipitate represented by (+) which is easily distinguished from fibrin strand precipitate or gel. Fibrinogen degradation products give no visible precipitate.

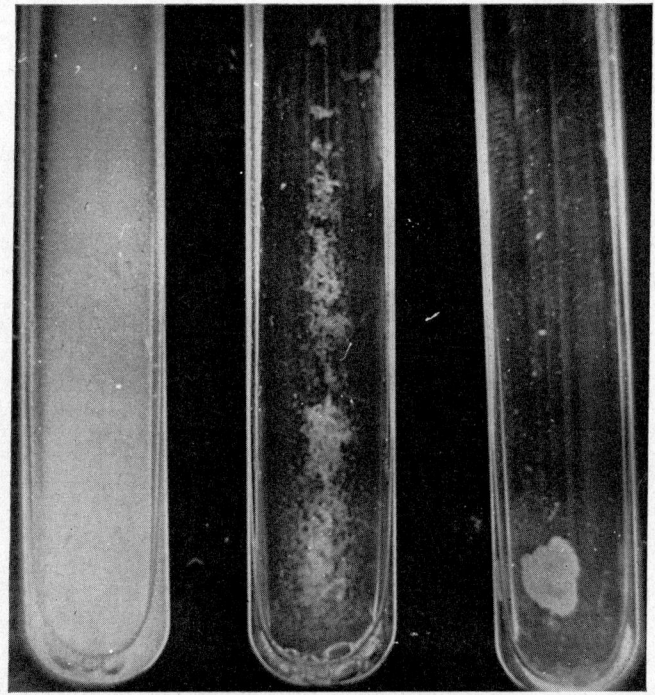

FIG. 4.2. SDPS precipitate—left: amorphous, fine granular precipitate formed with fibrin; centre: fibrin strands; right: gel which represents more advanced paracoagulation. From Niewiarowski, S. and Gurewich, V. (1971) *J. Lab. clin. Med*, **77**, 665–676.

Only fibrin strand precipitate or gel formation represents a positive test. The SDPS test is sensitive to less than 1 mg per cent fibrin monomers and less than 0·5 mg per cent early fibrin degradation products. The appearance of a positive precipitate is quite characteristic and easily recognised (Fig. 4.2). The amorphous, fine granular precipitate formed with fibrinogen is shown in the test tube on the left. Fibrin strands are seen in the middle test tube and a gel which represents a more advanced paracoagulation reaction is shown in the photograph on the right.

Niewiarowski, Stewart and Marder have shown that the polymerization of fibrin monomers and early fibrin degradation products after the addition of appropriate concentrations of protamine sulphate results in a polymer that is indistinguishable electronmicroscopically from fibrin which is formed through the interaction of thrombin and fibrinogen (Niewiarowski *et al.*, 1970). The SDPS test, therefore, appears to be quite specific for these two fibrinogen

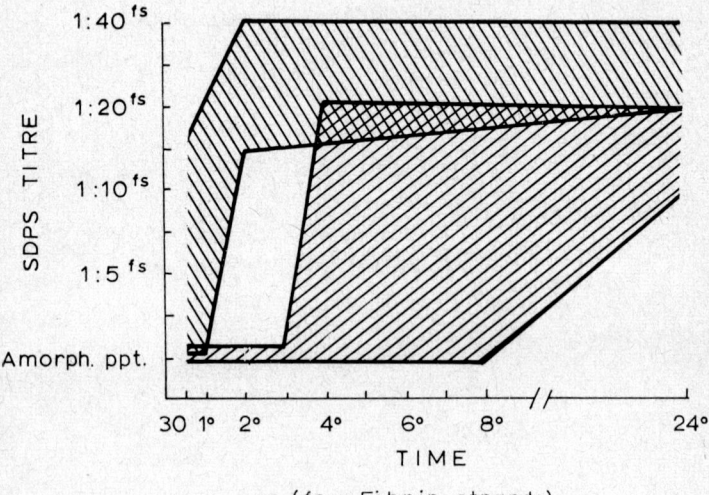

FIG. 4.3. Kinetics of PS-induced dissociation of fdp and FM complexes. From Gurewich, V., Niewiarowski, S. and Hutchinson, E. (1971) *Thrombos. Diathes. haemorrh.* (*Stuttg.*), Suppl.

derivatives. The 24 hour observation period enables a distinction to be made between fibrin monomers and early fibrin degradation products (Fig. 4.3). Under the conditions of the test, fibrin monomers tend to be dissociated from their complexes by protamine sulphate and polymerize to form a fibrin strand precipitate or gel within the first 30 to 60 minutes. In contrast, fibrin strand precipitate formation due to polymerization of early fibrin degradation products is delayed, often for 24 hours. The distinction between these two products is of practical importance in a number of clinical situations and opens the possibility to distinguish 'hypercoagulability' from overt thrombosis.

Although the serial dilution method makes the test semiquantitative, more precise quantitation is achieved by diluting out the test plasma with a 9:1 mixture of Tris buffer and 3·8 per cent sodium citrate (Table 4.2).

The SDPS test is then run on each plasma dilution and the last one giving a positive reaction is multiplied by the sensitivity of the test. The designation fy on the table stands for feathery precipitate which represents the lowest grade positive reaction.

TABLE 4.2

QUANTITATION TABLE

Dilutions of plasma containing 8 mg per cent FM made with Tris buffer (0·05M) and 3·8 per cent citrate (9:1).

Plasma dilutions	PS dilutions			
8 mg % FM	1:5	1:10	1:20	1:40
1: 1	g ++	g ++	g ++	g ++
1: 2	g ++	g ++	g ++	g +
1: 4	fs	fs	fs	fs
1: 8	fy	fy	—	—
1:16	—	—	—	—

Since the SDPS test is insensitive to fibrinogen degradation products, the test readily distinguishes primary from secondary fibrinolytic states. The elaboration of thrombin is required for a positive test to develop. When fibrinolytic agents such as streptokinase are administered, the SDPS test remains negative despite the generation of large amounts of fibrinogen degradation products. The test becomes positive, however, when fibrinolysis is achieved and fibrin degradation products are formed. The correlation between the development of a positive SDPS test during fibrinolytic therapy and angiographically proven lysis has been 100 per cent in our experience. These observations are illustrated by some animal experiments (Fig. 4.4). The effect of a 30 minute infusion of streptokinase into 6 rabbits resulted in fibrinogenolysis and a reduction in the amount of amorphous precipitate formed in the SDPS test. However, no positive reaction developed. When small amounts of thrombin (10 NIH units) were infused, a positive test due to the formation of fibrin monomers resulted. Fibrin deposition did not take place in these animals. A subsequent infusion of streptokinase resulted in a return to a negative reaction, presumably due to lysis of fibrin monomers. In the last group of animals, fresh thromboemboli were formed and released to the lungs. Ten minutes after embolization, a positive SDPS test was found in each animal. The subsequent administration of streptokinase resulted in a more positive test in 5 of the 6 animals and a continued positive reaction of the same titre in the 6th. These changes were associated with lysis of the thromboemboli and represent the appearance of fibrin degradation products in the circulation.

Our clinical experience with the SDPS test for the detection of intravascular coagulation has been encouraging. In 75 healthy subjects ranging in age from 18 to 75, the test was negative. Women

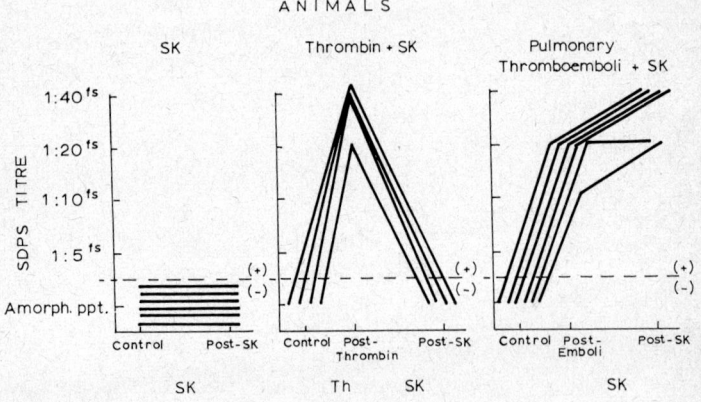

Fig. 4.4. The effects of streptokinase infusion into rabbits.

in the early menstrual phase of their ovarian cycle may have a slightly positive test which is negative during the remainder of the cycle. In 10 cases of well-documented disseminated intravascular coagulation, the SDPS test was strongly positive in each case.

In a number of conditions known to be associated with activated coagulation or thrombosis, a certain incidence of positive tests of varying magnitude has been found. These conditions include the post-operative state, pregnancy (but more particularly the immediate postpartum period), cirrhosis, acute pancreatitis and chronic renal failure. In 10 patients with documented acute pulmonary embolism the test was uniformly positive (Table 4.3).

Lung scans considered unequivocally indicative of pulmonary embolism were present in 9 of the patients and angiographic confirmation was obtained in 3 patients. The staphylococcal clumping test (SCT) which is a measure of fibrinogen-fibrin degradation products (Hawiger et al., 1970) was positive in each patient in whom it was performed. The normal titre is less than 1:4 and our finding of elevated titres of degradation products in pulmonary embolism confirms the experience first published by Ruckley et al. (1970) and more recently by Wilson et al. (1971). No false negatives have been encountered in either disseminated intravascular coagulation or pulmonary embolism.

TABLE 4.3

ACUTE PULMONARY THROMBOEMBOLISM

Sex and age	Underlying disease	X-ray	ECG	Lung scan	Angio	SDPS	SCT
M 74	CHF	Negative	RV strain	+		1: 5 fs	
F 32	Oral contraceptives	Effusion	Normal	+	+	1:40 fs	
F 50	Post-operative	Effusion	Normal	+	+	1:40 fs	
M 66	ASHD	Infiltrates	RV strain			1:20 g	1:16
F 87	CHF	Infiltrates	LVH	+		1: 5 fs	1:32
F 50	Metastatic cancer Post-operative	Effusion	Normal	+		1:40 fs	
F 25	Post-partum	Effusion Infiltrates	Normal	+		1:20 fs	
F 20	Oral contraceptives Thrombophlebitis	Negative	RV strain	+		1:40 g	1:256
M 66	Idiopathic	Effusion Infiltrates	RV strain	+	+	1:10 fy	1:32
M 66	Prostatic cancer Oestrogen Rx	Infiltrates		+		1:10 fs	1:4
						10/10	

After heparin treatment is initiated, the SDPS test gradually becomes negative, usually over a period of 48 to 72 hours. The test itself is not affected by heparin. This response is illustrated by the data on one of the patients with pulmonary embolism (Table 4.4).

The SDPS reactions, the last plasma dilution at which a positive reaction was found, SCT and lung scan results are shown. The increase in plasma dilution seen on the second day was probably due to lysis with release of fibrin degradation products into the circulation similar to what was seen in the animal experiments. The formation of a fibrin strand precipitate was delayed in this and subsequent samples, a finding characteristic of fibrin degradation products rather than fibrin monomers. Our experience with acute deep vein thrombosis is summarised (Table 4.5).

The clinical diagnosis in each of the 22 cases and based on the

TABLE 4.4
A CASE HISTORY

A 20 year-old female on oral contraceptives for 4 months. Pain and swelling left calf 23.2.71. Chest pain, syncope, SOB 1.3.71. Tachycardia, fixed split second heart sound, P2 . ECG: S1, Q3, T3, T $V_1 - V_3$. Chest X-ray: normal. Lung scan: several large defects. Marked clinical improvement by 3.3.71.

Date	1/3	2/3	3/3	4/3	5/3	8/3
Treatment	—	Heparin i.v. 10,000–7,000 u., 4 hourly					
SDPS	1:40 g	1:20 g	1:5 fs	neg	neg	neg
Plasma dilution	1:64	1:128	1:2	—	—	—
SCT	1:256	—	1:64	1:4	1:2	1:2
SCAN	POSITIVE				NEGATIVE	

presence of acute, unilateral swelling, tenderness, cyanosis and distention of the superficial venous system. Confirmation was obtained by the Doppler flow meter technique or by venography. The SDPS test was positive in 17 out of the 22 patients. In 12 patients in whom fibrinogen-fibrin degradation products were measured by the SCT, elevated levels were also found. This latter finding stands in contrast

TABLE 4.5
ACUTE DEEP VEIN THROMBOSIS

No. of patients	Doppler flow meter	Venogram	SDPS	SCT
22	16/16	13/3	17/22	12/12

to the finding of Wilson *et al.* (1971) who did not detect elevated titres of fibrinogen-fibrin degradation products, as measured by the tanned red cell technique, in deep vein thrombosis which was not accompanied by pulmonary embolism.

Some of the diagnostic findings from one of our patients with deep vein thrombosis and no evidence of pulmonary embolism are shown in Fig. 4.5. The venogram showed extensive femoral vein thrombosis. On the left is a photograph of the patient's SDPS test, namely the gel as it appeared in the test tube when the plasma was added to a 1:20 dilution of protamine sulphate. The electronmicroscopic structure of this gel is also shown and is a characteristic fibrin network.

In summary, the SDPS test represents a simple, sensitive and specific haematologic assay for two fibrinogen derivatives which are indicative of thrombosis. The test appears to be invariably positive in disseminated intravascular coagulation and acute pulmonary thromboembolism and is usually positive in deep vein thrombosis.

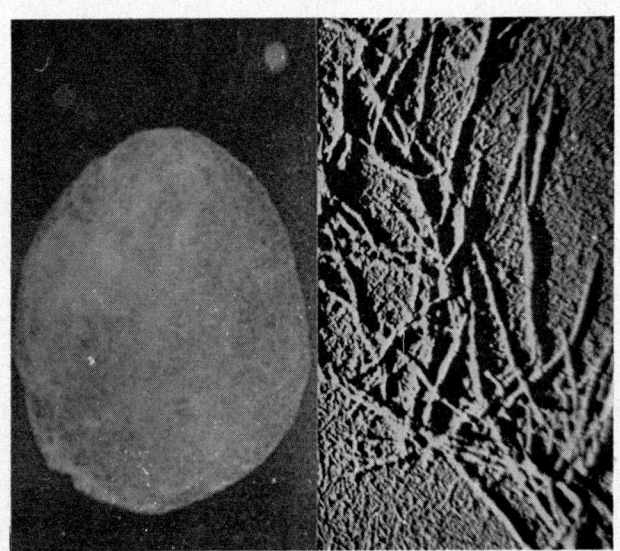

FIG. 4.5. Diagnostic findings in a patient with deep vein thrombosis. From Gurewich, V. and Hutchinson, E. (1971) *Annals int. Med.*, in press.

The SCT represents a useful corroborative assay which like the SDPS test is simple and requires no special equipment. The two tests differ from each other in that the SDPS test is insensitive to fibrinogen degradation products and specifically identifies fibrin degradation products. This allows it to be used as a haematologic measure of efficacy in thrombolytic therapy.

REFERENCES

DERECHIN, M. (1955) *Rev. Hémat.*, **10,** 41.
HAWIGER, J. *et al.* (1970) *J. Lab. clin. Med.*, **75,** 93.
KOPEC, M. *et al.* (1962) *Thrombos. Diathes. haemorrh (Stuttg.)*, **5,** 285.
NIEWIAROWSKI, S. *et al.*(1970) *Biochim. biophys. Acta (Amst.)*, **221,** 326.
NIEWIAROWSKI, S. and GUREWICH, V. (1971) *J. Lab. clin. Med.*, **77,** 665.
RUCKLEY, C. V. *et al.* (1970) *Brit. med. J.* **4,** 395.
WILSON, J. E. III *et al.* (1971) *J. clin. Invest.* **50,** 474.

5 Discussion

Le Quesne: Could Dr. Flute say what number of his patients received Macrodex; his conclusions refer to the changes in blood of patients undergoing an operation, but it seems that the changes seen are those in patients having and operation plus Macrodex. Dr. Flute has said there is no correlation between platelet stickiness and the development of deep vein thrombosis, but earlier he indicated that most of the patients had received Macrodex, which alters platelet stickiness.

Flute: This is a valid comment. Not all the negative results have been presented. We looked carefully and found no difference between patients receiving Macrodex and the others for fibrinogen, fibrin degradation products or dilute clot lysis time. The only positive difference was in platelet adhesiveness using the Hellem technique.

Perhaps our numbers are too few to allow correlation between a change in adhesiveness and the development of deep vein thrombosis.

Thomas: Could Dr. Flute suggest why FDP levels go up in patients with thromboembolism? Why should the presence of an embolus in the lung, or its move from the leg to the lung, cause a large rise in the level of FDPs?

Flute: Are they fibrin degradation products? Assuming so, they may be related to tissue damage, though the deep veins in the leg and the lung, with its two circulations, are not really grossly damaged. The level of fibrin degradation products is similar to that observed in patients treated with streptokinase.

Barkhan: The lung is rich in plasminogen activator, and the presence of an embolus may stimulate release of activator from the pulmonary vessels.

Thomas: Wilson, in Dallas, Texas, using the Merskey technique of measuring FDP, has found high levels within an hour or two of embolism. Whether these levels were also present before the embolism is not known, but it would suggest that fibrin degradation products are formed in association with embolisation.

Flute: We have studied patients at daily intervals before embolism; there was no evidence of an increase in general fibrinolysis sufficient to produce such changes.

Sherry: The impaction of fibrin in the pulmonary vascular bed is no different from its impaction in the microcirculation in other areas. It usually results in active local fibrinolysis; thus, an increase in local fibrinolysis after pulmonary embolism is to be expected.

There is ample evidence that the microcirculation is much richer in fibrinolytic activity than the systemic circulation; probably it is the source of most of the plasma activator. Furthermore, there is evidence to suggest that endothelial cells continuously secrete small amounts of activator into the local circulation.

Ruckley: We have demonstrated high levels of FDPs in the venous drainage of legs which are the site of acute arterial occlusion, a finding which is in agreement with Professor Sherry's comments.

Dr. Flute cannot assume that the ^{125}I-fibrinogen test will distinguish patients with deep vein thrombosis. This technique separates patients who have venous thrombosis below the level of the inguinal ligament from those who have not.

Flute: Yes—'deep vein thrombosis of the leg' is perhaps too wide a statement. However, the changes of major thrombosis involving vessels above the inguinal ligament almost certainly will be evident clinically.

Johnson: The increase in FDPs was moderate in the majority of about 50 patients in the United States pulmonary embolism trial. High levels were found in 6 only.

Sherry: More attention should be paid to the equilibrium state; activators are likely to be balanced by inhibitors. When considering hypercoagulability, attention has been focussed on the identification of changes in coagulation factors or the presence of activators. Investigation into a possible deficiency of inhibitors might well identify the thrombosis-prone individual.

In a patient stressed by surgery or local trauma, there is local deposition of fibrin. Thrombin, or earlier activated components which leak to the general circulation, require inactivation by, for example, anti-thrombin. It should be possible to demonstrate a progressive decrease in the level of anti-thrombin III or associated substances. Is there any evidence that stressed patients with local trauma and local fibrin formation have a progressive diminution in the levels of inhibitors to the coagulation mechanism?

Wessler: This has been claimed for anti-thrombin III. We have not studied patients yet because our work has been concentrated on the animal model.

An increase, rather than a decrease, in inhibitor should be sought. We have evidence that heparin is a profound stimulus to an apparent increase in inhibitor activity. Intravascular coagulation may result in the release of small amounts of heparin, which is the factor measured.

Sherry: It might be more appropriate to identify the protein component itself. It is possible to develop an immuno-assay for antithrombin III?

Wessler: Yes it is. However, it would still be necessary to know what was being measured by immuno-assay and whether biological activity were present.

Barkhan: Does the curve which Dr. Fletcher showed alter post-operatively due to the presence of haemostatic thrombi?

Fletcher: Data were obtained for 6 samples (pre-operative, one hour post-operative, and the succeeding four days) for each of 19 patients who developed deep vein thrombosis and 12 who did not.

Pre-operatively, there was no difference in the amount of polymer —4 per cent and 8 per cent respectively.

One hour post-operatively, there was a marked difference (18 per cent compared with 2 per cent) in the group of patients who later developed thrombosis. Most thrombi were diagnosed on the first post-operative day, when the difference—41 per cent compared with 12 per cent—was equally striking. On the fourth day, the level was normal in the patients without thrombi, but 31 per cent in those with, the reason being that the thrombi were still present in these patients.

In both groups there was a rise in fibrinogen first derivative during operation which remained elevated for 5 days.

The shift to the left is meaningful and we do not make a diagnosis of thrombosis unless there is more than 20 per cent polymer.

Gurewich: Our findings are similar. There is a high incidence in the early post-operative period (the first 5 days) of positive tests. In those patients who do not develop post-operative deep vein thrombosis, the levels are relatively low. Since the test is semi-quantitative we are attempting to establish the normal post-operative range.

In an extensive study of post-partum patients, there is a similar pattern, all patients having a positive test. But those who develop thrombo-embolic complications have higher initial titres and remain positive longer.

Sherry: Since the first derivative of fibrin proteolysis reacts in this paracoagulation scheme, why doesn't the first derivative of fibrinogen proteolysis, particularly since the latter is a clottable protein?

Gurewich: Both fibrin monomer and fibrin degradation products do react. With fibrinogen degradation products, the electron microscope reveals small strands.

Flute: There is some difficulty in reading the end-point with the test described by Dr. Gurewich. In a blind study, we have tested female patients three times pre-operatively, immediately after operation, on the first post-operative day, on an intermediate day and then on the sixth day.

The pre-operative results show a small scatter. There was a great increase in the number of positives after operation. The test was strongly positive in all 5 patients who developed deep vein thrombosis; of the 28 patients who did not have a detectable thrombus (using the labelled fibrinogen technique and sometimes venography), 23 were also positive.

I suggest that the results of these tests are due to surgery rather than thrombosis. Is Dr. Fletcher certain that his patients had similarly severe operations?

Fletcher: The majority had operations described as major by the surgeons—being mostly thoracic cases.

The protamine test has been in use for about 15 years and it has been modified frequently. We use Latallo's modification and have found some degree of correlation with our chromatographic results. Roughly, in 70 per cent of patients with more than 20 per cent polymer, the protamine test is positive. Further work is needed to improve on the 30 per cent false positives.

Gaffney: How are fibrin degradation products distinguished from fibrinogen degradation products, from a molecular point of view, by Dr. Gurewich's test?

Gurewich: The SPDS test is more sensitive than previous protamine sulphate tests. Although a wide variety of diseases give positive results, a negative test is useful because it can be used to exclude the presence of a pulmonary embolus. Most of the differential diagnoses (e.g. pneumonia or congestive cardiac failure) give a negative result.

The difference between fibrinogen and fibrin degradation products is that the polypeptide chain has been removed from early fibrin degradation products and this allows para-coagulation.

Sherry: These tests seem to imply that, when positive, there is a thrombus present. However, does a negative test in a patient with

DISCUSSION

pneumonia or heart failure mean the absence of and a positive test the presence of, an intravascular thrombus?

Gurewich: These tests do not reflect the presence of a thrombus. I believe they show hypercoagulability. In the experimental animal, an infusion of small amounts of thrombin causes a positive test, but no fibrin deposition is observed under the microscope. Probably only fibrin monomer is formed in the circulation, without going on to polymerization, thus representing changes which precede thrombus formation.

In the presence of a thrombus, the test will also be positive by detecting either fibrin precursor or products of lysis initiated by thrombus formation.

Thus, it is possible that the test will enable the initiation of therapy before a thrombotic event has occurred.

Fletcher: When a thrombus is detected by the ^{125}I-fibrinogen technique, its resolution can be followed; data from the chromatographic method is in accord.

Our findings on the arterial side are interesting. In cerebrovascular thrombosis, the chromatographic technique has been useful prognostically. Patients with an incomplete lesion who show a lytic pattern, recover well; those with severely abnormal patterns do badly. However, a middle cerebral artery thrombus is small; are the changes detected a reflection of hypercoagulability and is the patient's outlook dependent on this?

Widmer: The ^{125}I-fibrinogen technique has its limitations. I would propose a search for new tests of hypercoagulability and their correlation with venography.

Kakkar: We have been giving low doses of subcutaneous heparin in an attempt to prevent deep vein thrombosis in a group of hernia patients. In the controls, the incidence of venous thrombosis, using the radioisotope method, was 24 per cent. In the patients receiving heparin, the incidence was reduced to 4 per cent. Can Professor Wessler explain these findings?

Wessler: Your results are those we would hope for if our concept of the coagulation sequence is valid. Once Factor X is activated, the sequence is fast. The action of heparin is directed primarily towards increasing the activity of the inhibitor to activated factor X; thus heparin, given early, should be effective, even in doses which do not affect the clotting time. More heparin is needed if thrombosis is occurring, as is shown by clinical experience in the therapy of pulmonary emboli—more units of heparin are needed at the onset of heparin therapy than are required one week later when intravascular coagulation has subsided.

If your data can be correlated with the levels of heparin, it might be possible to give heparin at a dose that will not interfere with haemostasis and would still be antithrombotic.

PART II
PREVENTION AND DIAGNOSIS

6 The Dynamics of Venous Blood Flow and the Prevention of Deep Venous Thrombosis

L. T. Cotton, S. Sabri and V. C. Roberts

INTRODUCTION

Since the first description of a case of post-operative deep vein thrombosis (Strauch, 1894), the mortality rate of thromboembolism has continued to rise at an alarming rate. The deaths recorded in the Registrar General's Report for England and Wales from 1943 to 1969 have been plotted in Fig. 6.1. Assuming that the present trend continues, then extrapolation of the curves to the year 1973 indicates that there will have been a tenfold increase in mortality over a period of 30 years. Whatever may have been the cause of this increase in mortality, we believe that there can be no doubt that it is a genuine increase, and not due merely to increased awareness or to improved methods of diagnosis.

It has been against this background of such an alarming increase in thromboembolism that this present study into the causes of deep venous thrombosis has been carried out. It represents several years of efforts by a team of surgeons and engineers who have been looking at blood flow from a mechanical and physiopathological point of view. The role of engineering in this field has been vital since the measurement and analysis of venous blood flow patterns are a mechanical problem and particularly suitable for study by engineers.

Rudolf Virchow, with the greatest foresight, wrote in 1856 that a principal cause of thrombosis was slowing of blood flow. However, this was followed by a period during which platelet activity and other haematological factors were considered to be the determinant causes (Rokitansky, 1852; Zahn, 1875; Bizzozero, 1882; Welsh, 1887; Eberth and Schimmelbusch, 1888; Aschoff, 1924; and Wright, 1942), and it has taken over a hundred years for us to come a full circle and realise how prophetic was his original statement. Now that stagnation of venous blood flow is being studied as a prime cause of thrombosis, results are coming fast—not only in terms of the anatomical localisation of thrombi but, far more important, the means of preventing them.

The recent developments in this field indicate that Virchow was absolutely right in his hypothesis that stasis is the all important

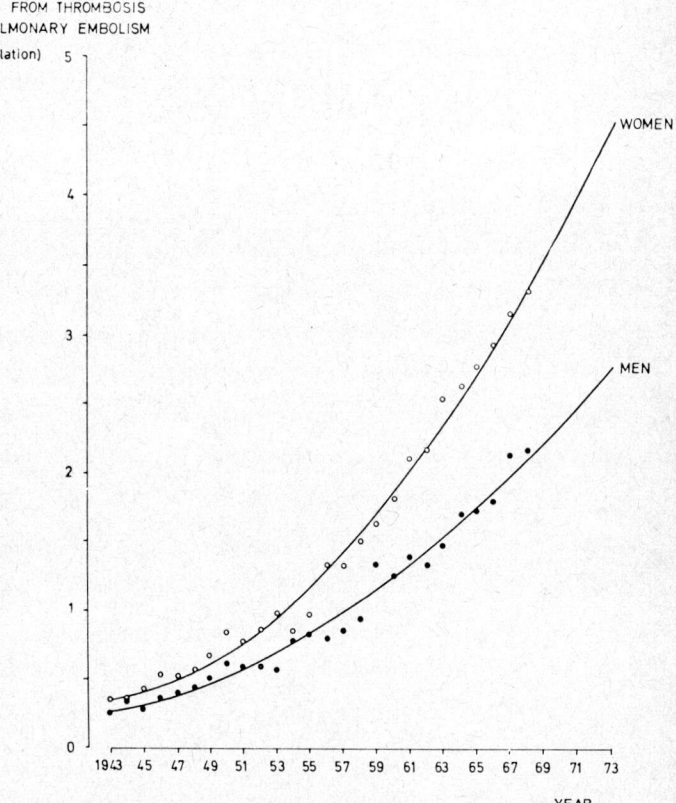

FIG. 6.1. The rising mortality rate from thromboembolism.

factor producing venous thrombosis. It is natural, therefore, to suggest that the way to prevent thrombosis is to promote venous blood flow, particularly during operations. It would perhaps, be preferable, to prevent deep venous thrombosis by the administration of some drug, but at present it seems that effective, practical, prophylaxis will require the application to the legs, of machines designed to assist the venous return.

ANATOMICAL LOCALISATION OF VENOUS THROMBOSIS

The first really detailed analysis of the sites of deep venous thrombosis in the leg were reported by Gibbs (1957). He dissected the legs of 239 cadavers and found thrombosis in 124 patients. He

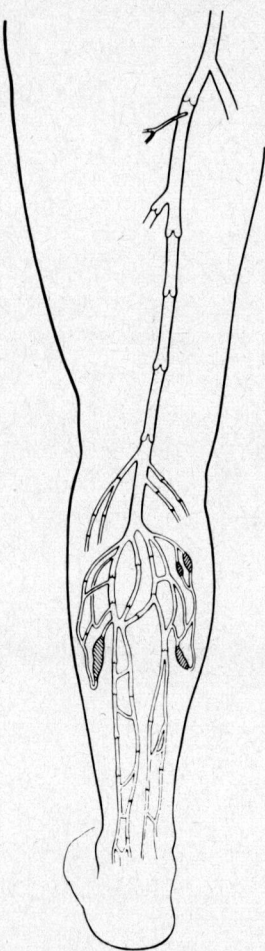

Fig. 6.2. The soleal sinuses.

then classified the sites of thrombosis and found the commonest site by far to be in the veins of the soleus muscles. The soleal sinuses (Fig. 6.2) are an essential part of the pumping mechanism that allows us to stand on our hind legs for they form the chambers of the peripheral heart that propel blood from the feet to the heart when we are standing and during exercise. As far as we know they are unique to man. More recent work has confirmed that it is in the soleal sinuses that the vast majority of deep vein thromboses arise (Cotton and Clark, 1965). It seems that during surgery the soleal sinuses become foci of venous stasis and later thrombosis.

MEASUREMENT OF VENOUS BLOOD FLOW DURING SURGERY

Our group was the first to measure venous blood flow rate directly in the femoral and iliac veins during surgery. These measurements were carried out using the principle of thermal dilution (Clark and Cotton, 1968; Clark, 1968). This involved the use of a minute probe mounted on the end of a long, fine nylon catheter which was inserted into a major vein draining a leg. During use, saline at room temperature is injected through the probe and sprays out retrogradely into the oncoming venous blood stream, through four fine orifices bored in the centre of the probe. A thermistor mounted inside the middle of the probe measures the temperature of the saline before it leaves the probe; another thermistor mounted on the tip of the probe measures the temperature of the mixture of blood and saline as it flows past the probe. From these two temperatures the mass blood flow rate can be estimated continuously.

Fifteen patients having a variety of operations were studied and the outstanding conclusion was that venous flow rates were remarkably depressed, especially at the beginning of an operation. In a typical patient, flow measured in the external iliac vein fell by 50 per cent when anaesthesia was induced with thiopentone sodium—a fall which was, moreover, maintained. If this degree of change is produced in the iliac veins then it can reasonably be concluded that the flow in the soleal sinuses will be similarly or even more reduced.

It is on this fall of venous flow during surgery that our efforts have been concentrated during the last few years; the effects of mechanical methods of increasing both the venous return and the pulsatility of the venous flow waveform have been studied in detail. There have been many attempts in recent years at prevention of deep venous thrombosis during surgery by such techniques as bandaging or elevation of the legs and electrical stimulation of the calf muscles. However, we decided from the outset that we would not try any mechanical method to prevent deep venous thrombosis until we had found out exactly what each did to venous blood flow.

Venous blood flow in the femoral vein has now been measured in 50 patients during varicose vein surgery. During these operations electromagnetic flow meter probes have been placed around the common femoral veins after division of the saphenofemoral junction. Both veins have been exposed so that one can be used as a control while conducting an investigation on the other.

EFFECT OF EXTERNAL APPLICATION OF STATIC PRESSURE ON FEMORAL VEIN FLOW

Increments of static pressure were uniformly applied to the leg by means of an inflatable splint (Parke Davis and Co.). Femoral venous flow was measured at each increment of pressure (Fig. 6.3). At low pressures there is a small but significant rise in the flow in both the compressed and control legs (Spiro *et al.*, 1970; Sabri *et al.*, 1971a) but, as the pressure rises the flow is progressively reduced.

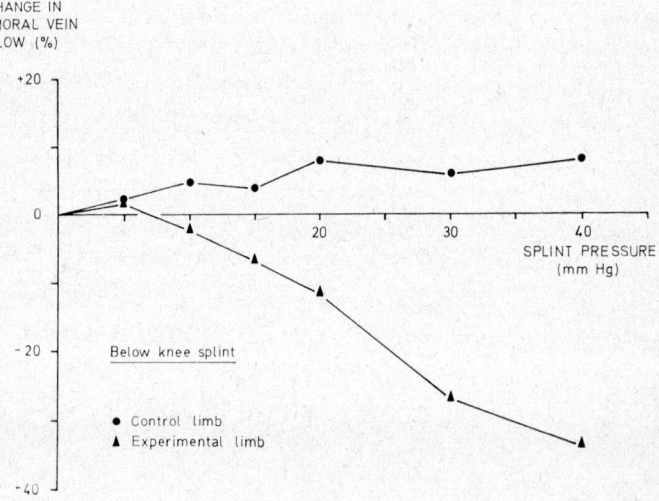

FIG. 6.3. Femoral venous flow.

At a pressure of 40 mm Hg the flow measured at the groin is reduced by almost 40 per cent; presumably at the level of the calf the reduction in flow would be even greater.

In order to correlate these results with the effects of bandaging we enlisted the help of a group of 22 nurses. They were asked to bandage a subject's leg first with a crepe bandage and then, after removing the crepe, a Bisgaard bandage was applied. The compression pressures produced by these bandages were measured with a special transducer. The results, shown in Table 6.1, indicate that the pressures produced by crepe bandages were fairly uniform, the mean value being about 13 mm Hg. However, with a Bisgaard bandage the mean pressure was 24 mm Hg and pressures in excess of 40 mm Hg (at which level flow can be seriously impaired) were recorded. Since performing these experiments we have stopped using Bisgaard bandages except in ambulant patients.

If then, it is important to increase venous blood flow to prevent deep venous thrombosis, bandaging would seem to offer little as a potential prophylactic. A recently conducted trial by Rosengarten et al. (1970) has indeed proved that bandaging the leg is ineffective in preventing deep venous thrombosis.

TABLE 6.1

COMPRESSION PRESSURES ACHIEVED BY A GROUP OF 22 NURSES USING CREPE AND BISGAARD BANDAGES

	Bandaging pressure (mm Hg)						
Bandage	0–6	6–12	12–18	18–24	24–30	30–36	36–42
Crepe	1	11	6	3	1	0	0
Bisgaard	1	0	5	5	6	2	3

PASSIVE EXERCISE DURING SURGERY

The best way of increasing blood flow to a limb is to exercise it. During surgery active exercise can only be achieved by electrical stimulation of the calf muscles, a prophylactic technique first advocated by Doran and his colleagues (1964). However, electrical stimulation has its drawbacks; it is difficult to control with any precision, its effects vary with the type of anaesthesia and erythema and blistering can sometime result. Furthermore, it does not lend itself easily to haemodynamic investigation.

An investigation has therefore been conducted into the effects of passive exercise during surgery using a motorised foot mover (Roberts et al., 1971). This foot mover consists essentially of a foot board, pivoted at the ankle which can be made to rock to and fro by means of an electric motor.

In the first part of the investigation, the effect of varying the rate of foot pedalling on the mean femoral venous flow rate was measured. In Fig. 6.4A is plotted the increase in femoral flow produced by passive exercise, as a function of the period of oscillation. As might be expected the faster the foot is moved (i.e. the smaller the period) the greater is the increase in the venous flow. The arterial inflow to the limb has also been measured and has been shown to increase similarly (Sabri et al., 1971b). Extrapolation of the mean flow increase back to zero shows that there will be no increase in venous flow if the period of oscillation is extended to about four seconds (Roberts et al., 1971). This may in part explain why some have been more successful than others in finding electrical stimulation an effective prophylactic.

The effect of passive exercise is not only to increase the mean venous flow but also to increase its pulsatility or the amplitude of the

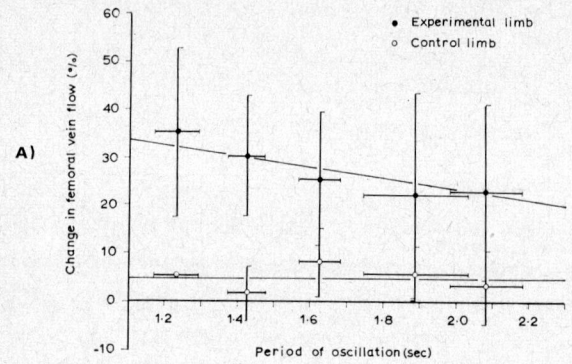

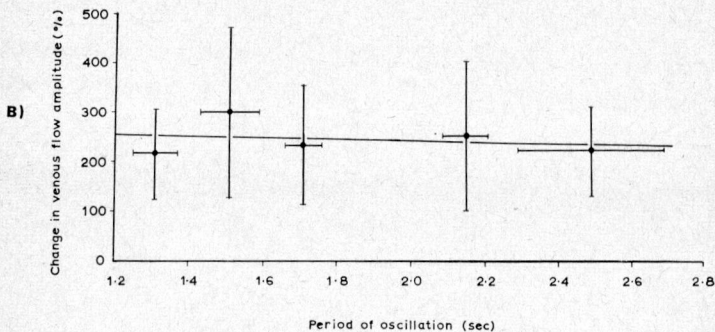

FIG. 6.4. Effects of passive exercise.

flow waveform. The results plotted in Fig. 6.4B show the increase in pulsatility is substantially independent of the period of oscillation of the foot whereas Fig. 6.5 shows that it very much depends on the degree to which the foot is moved, the maximal pulsatility being achieved when the foot is moved $\pm 30°$ to the vertical.

FOOT PEDALLING AND PREVENTION OF DEEP VENOUS THROMBOSIS

So impressive were the haemodynamics of passive exercise that a controlled trial was run to assess its potential value in preventing

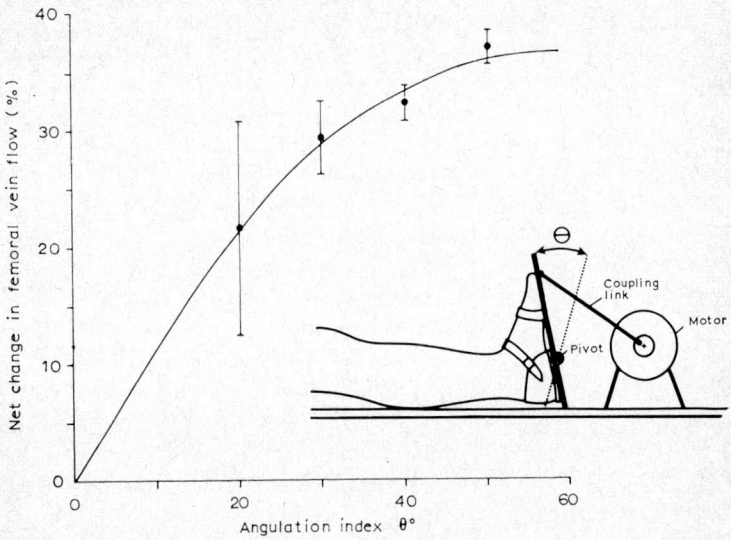

Fig. 6.5. Effect of angulation.

deep venous thrombosis. For the trial a random group of surgical patients aged 40 years or more were used and the presence of thrombosis was detected by the ^{125}I-fibrinogen test. In this trial each patient had only one leg pedalled and so each acted as his own control. The leg to be pedalled was decided by drawing a card from a pack. Using a sequential analysis we required only 47 patients to cross the line of 5 per cent significance. Out of these, eleven developed thrombi in the unpedalled leg alone and there was one in the pedalled leg alone. Two patients developed thrombi bilaterally. Thus passive exercise during surgery reduces the incidence of early post-operative deep venous thrombosis by 77 per cent.

INTERMITTENT COMPRESSION OF THE LEG

It has now been demonstrated that the incidence of DVT can be reduced by a method that increases both the mean level of venous flow and also its pulsatility. The question now to be answered is which is the more important? Our original investigation into the effects of static compression showed that, as pressure was applied to the leg, the venous flow rate rose transiently and then fell to a new level which was maintained so long as the static pressure was maintained.

From these results it has been possible to estimate the volume of blood which can be ejected from the leg by the application of an

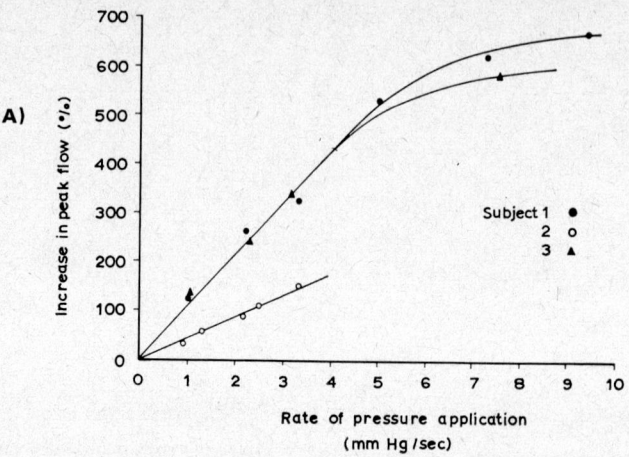

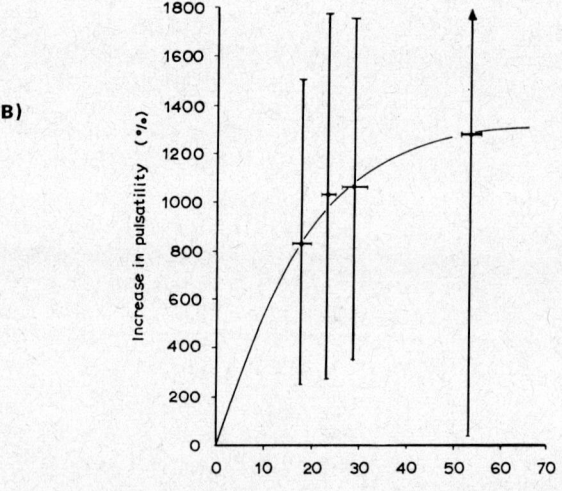

Fig. 6.6. Intermittent compression of the leg.

external pressure. It has been shown that the volume of venous blood squeezed out of the leg reaches a maximum when the applied pressure is about 30 mm Hg using a below-knee splint (Roberts, 1971).

The volume of blood that can be ejected from the calf is fixed for any given patient; thus, the peak flow achieved during compression must depend on how fast the compression is applied. The faster the leg is squeezed the greater is the peak flow. In Fig. 6.6A is plotted the rate of increasing pressure against the increase in the peak venous flow. The relationship is almost linear to 4 mm Hg per second and appears to be maximal at 8 mm Hg per second.

It appears therefore that, if the calf is compressed uniformly at a rate of 8 mm Hg per second up to a maximum pressure of 40 mm Hg, the venous system of the calf will have been emptied most rapidly, i.e. the maximum outflow will have been achieved in the minimum time. Any more prolonged compression is unnecessary and will only impair the general perfusion of the limb. If the compression is now

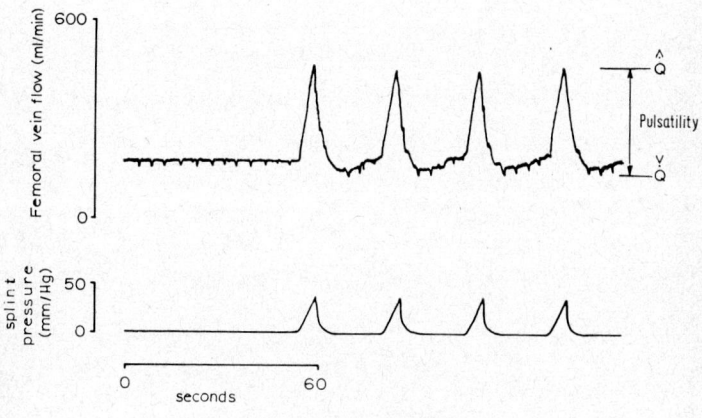

FIG. 6.7. Flow tracing.

released, the venous system will refill and the flow return to its resting level again. This process of refilling takes about one minute in unconscious patients. In Fig. 6.6B the increase in pulsatility produced by intermittent compression is plotted as a function of the interval between successive compressions, and as can be seen the effect is maximal when the interval is about one minute.

Maximal pulsatility of venous blood flow is achieved by compressive impulses rising at a rate of 8 mm Hg per second to 40 mm Hg at one minute intervals. Using these parameters we can increase the peak venous flow up to 700 per cent and the pulsatility can be increased thirty fold. A typical flow tracing is shown in Fig. 6.7. The mean venous flow is largely unchanged; thus, we have the means of determining whether increasing the pulsatility of venous flow is more important than increasing the mean flow rate.

INTERMITTENT COMPRESSION AND PREVENTION OF DEEP VENOUS THROMBOSIS

A trial of intermittent compression as a method of preventing deep venous thrombosis has recently been conducted using a machine that increased the pressure around the leg in the way described above. The trial was designed in the same way as that for the foot mover, and one leg was again used as control. Using the method of sequential statistical analysis the line of 5 per cent significance was crossed with only 39 patients. Eleven thrombi developed in the control legs (28·2 per cent), two occurred in the compressed legs, and of these one was bilateral. Thus intermittent compression reduced the incidence of deep venous thrombosis by 82 per cent.

CONCLUSION

Our results show that increasing the pulsatility of blood flow in the leg is the best method so far tried in the prevention of deep venous thrombosis. It is certainly the least troublesome logistically and we are encouraged to proceed to a major therapeutic trial of the method.

We would stress how much this project has only been possible by team work between surgeons and engineers—an example of the value of biomedical engineering.

REFERENCES

Aschoff, L. (1924) *Lectures on Pathology*, New York: Hoeber.
Bizzozero, J. (1882) *Virchows Arch. Path. Anat.*, **90,** 261.
Clark, C. (1968) *Med. and Biol. Engng.*, **6,** 133.
Clark, C. and Cotton, L. T. (1968) *Brit. J. Surg.*, **55,** 211.
Cotton, L. T. and Clark, C. (1965) *Ann. Roy. Coll. Surg. England*, **36,** 214.
Doran, F. S. A. et al. (1964) *Brit. J. Surg.*, **51,** 486.
Eberth, C. J. and Schimmelbusch, C. (1888) *Thrombose nach versuchen und leichenbefunden.* Stuttgart: E.M.K.E.
Gibbs, N. M. (1957) *Brit. J. Surg.*, **45,** 209.
Roberts, V. C. (1971) *Lancet*, **1,** 136.
Roberts, V. C. et al. (1970) *Brit. med. J.*, **4,** 556.
Roberts, V. C. et al. (1971) *Brit. med. J.*, **3,** 78.
Rokitansky, V. C. (1852) *A manual of Pathological Anatomy IV*, p. 336. London: Sydenham Society.
Rosengarten, D. S. (1970) *Brit. J. Surg.*, **57,** 296.
Sabri, S. et al. (1971a) *Brit. med. J.*, **3,** 503.
Sabri, S. et al. (1971b) *Cardiovasc. Res.*, in press.
Spiro, M. et al. (1970) *Brit. Med. J.*, **1,** 719.
Strauch, M. V. (1894) *Gymak*, **18,** 304.

WELSH, W. H. (1887) Reprinted in *William Henry Welsh. Papers and addresses*, vol. 1, p. 47. Baltimore: Johns Hopkins Press.
WRIGHT, H. P. (1942) *J. Path. Bact.*, **54**, 461.
ZAHN, F. W. (1875) *Virchows Arch. Path. Anat. Physiol.*, **62**, 81.

7 Soleal Veins, Stasis and Prevention of Deep Vein Thrombosis

A. N. Nicolaides, V. V. Kakkar, E. S. Field and P. Fish

INTRODUCTION

Recent investigations using the ^{125}I-fibrinogen test (Atkins and Hawkins, 1965; Flanc et al., 1968; Negus et al., 1968; Kakkar et al., 1970) have shown that the incidence of deep vein thrombosis is high, not only in general surgical patients (30 per cent—Flanc et al., 1968), but also in gynaecological (18 per cent—Friend, 1971), orthopaedic (50 per cent—Field et al., 1971) and urological patients (28 per cent—Nicolaides et al., 1972). In all these patients practically all thrombi had started in the calf. Studies with the ^{125}I-fibrinogen test have also demonstrated that in surgical patients 50 per cent of the thrombi start during the operation (Flanc et al., 1968) and that another 30 per cent during the subsequent 48 hours (Nicolaides, 1971d). The majority of these thrombi are harmless because they do not produce emboli; they either remain localised in the calf or lyse spontaneously (Kakkar et al., 1969). Twenty per cent, however, extend proximally into and above the popliteal vein and are then liable to break off and become emboli. It has been estimated that when they extend into the pelvic veins the incidence of pulmonary embolism becomes approximately 50 per cent (Kakkar et al., 1969).

The fact that thrombi start in the calf at the time of operation or soon after means that the factors responsible for intravascular coagulation produce their maximum effect there at this particular time. *In vitro* experiments have shown that, immediately after injury, contact factors are found circulating in the blood in an activated form (Penick et al., 1965). The production of thrombi has been shown to depend on the presence of such activated factors in an area of stasis (Wessler and Yin, 1968). Thrombosis, however, is not produced by stasis alone or by activated factors alone, but by the combination of the two (Wessler and Yin, 1968).

It has already been demonstrated that stasis which occurs in the valve pockets and in the muscular veins of the calf in conscious patients, can be reduced by leg elevation and exercises (McLachin et al., 1960). Several attempts to prevent deep vein thrombosis by preventing stasis in trials where the patients were screened with the ^{125}I-fibrinogen test have been reported recently. Simple measures such as leg elevation (Rosengarten and Laird, 1971), elastic stockings alone (Rosengarten et al., 1970) or in combination with leg exercises (Flanc et al., 1969) have been ineffective. Electric stimulation of the calf muscles during operation has produced a 61 per cent relative reduction in the incidence of deep vein thrombosis (Browse and Negus, 1970), but this has not been confirmed by subsequent workers (De Jode et al., 1970). Passive exercise of the leg during surgery using a motorised foot mover has produced a 77 per cent relative reduction in the incidence of deep vein thrombosis (Sabri et al., 1971), but unfortunately this study was limited to the first three days after operation. Intermittent calf compression using pneumatic leggings has also reduced the incidence of post-operative deep vein thrombosis by 66 per cent (Hills et al., 1971).

The purpose of the present study was to determine the exact site in the calf where thrombi start; to determine the degree of stasis in the veins of the calf and particularly the soleal veins not only in conscious but also in anaesthetised patients during operation. An attempt has also been made to evaluate the effect of various methods to prevent stasis with the view of eventually using the most effective one in a clinical trial.

MATERIAL AND METHODS

The investigation was divided in six parts:

1. SITE OF ORIGIN OF DEEP VEIN THROMBI

Method: A technique of venography has been used which consistently demonstrates the soleal veins in addition to the other deep veins of the leg up to the inferior vena cava. This has been described in detail elsewhere (Nicolaides et al., 1971c). Briefly, the patient lies horizontal on the X-ray table. A scalp vein infusion needle is introduced into a vein on the dorsum of the foot. A 5 cm-wide pneumatic cuff is placed at the ankle to prevent any filling of the superficial veins and a similar mid-thigh cuff to occlude the femoral vein. The veins of the leg are first partially emptied either by a lightly applied elastic crepe bandage or by leg elevation. The ankle cuff is then inflated to 120 mm Hg and the mid-thigh cuff to 200 mm Hg. This does not occlude the arterial blood flow because of the narrowness of the cuff. The injection of 45 per cent sodium diatrizoate (Hypaque) is commenced, the bandage is removed and the leg is returned to the horizontal position. The contrast medium is seen on the image intensifier to ascend in the tibial veins and to fill the soleal veins in a retrograde fashion. After taking films of the leg in two planes and of the popliteal and lower femoral veins, the mid-thigh cuff is released, the injection is continued and films are taken of the upper femoral and pelvic veins. A total of 60–80 ml of contrast medium is injected. At the end of the examination the cuffs are removed and the veins are cleared of contrast medium by leg elevation assisted by injecting 150 ml of normal saline containing 2500 units of heparin. Complete clearance is confirmed by fluoroscopy of the leg.

The diagnosis of a thrombus is made when a constant filling defect is seen on at least two films. Non-visualisation of a vein is not considered diagnostic of thrombosis unless there is good opacification proximally and distally with the presence of a collateral circulation (De Weese and Rogoff, 1963; Nicolaides, 1971c).

Selection of patients: The technique described above has been used in 121 consecutive patients referred to the Department of Surgery because of clinically suspected acute deep vein thrombosis. Venography performed within hours was used to prove or disprove the presence of thrombi. Eleven patients had massive thrombosis with oedema up to the groin, while in the remaining 110 patients the clinical signs were confined below the knee.

2. CLEARANCE OF SODIUM DIATRIZOATE FROM TIBIAL AND SOLEAL VEINS

Method: The technique of venography described above has been used to fill the soleal and tibial veins. After injecting 30 ml of 45 per cent sodium diatrizoate and filling the soleal and tibial veins, the injection is stopped, the mid-thigh cuff is removed and the time taken by the contrast medium to disappear from the soleal and tibial veins is measured using a stopwatch (Nicolaides *et al.*, 1971b).

Selection of patients: The clearance times of sodium diatrizoate from the tibial and soleal veins have been determined in 46 conscious patients who were found to have normal veins during the course of venography. Venography was performed in these patients in order to prove or disprove the clinical diagnosis of deep vein thrombosis. Patients with thrombi, oedema or cellutitis were excluded. The clearance times have been determined when the leg was horizontal (16 patients), when the leg was horizontal but with a full-length elastic stocking on (5 patients), when the leg was elevated 20° (10 patients), during active plantar flexion of the foot

(5 patients), during electric stimulation of the calf muscles (5 patients) and during active plantar flexion of the foot against resistance (5 patients). (Nicolaides et al., 1971b).

3. SIMULTANEOUS CLEARANCE OF SODIUM DIATRIZOATE AND ^{125}I-FIBRINOGEN FROM SOLEAL AND TIBIAL VEINS

Method: Exactly the same technique has been used to direct the contrast medium into the tibial and soleal veins as described above, but 10 μCi of ^{125}I-fibrinogen were added to the 30 ml of 45 per cent sodium diatrizoate injected. The thyroid of the patients had already been blocked with sodium iodide (100 mg orally) as part of the routine screening with the ^{125}I-fibrinogen test. After releasing the mid-thigh cuff a clearance curve of the ^{125}I-fibrinogen from the calf was obtained while the disappearance of the sodium diatrizoate as seen on the image intensifier was timed. The clearance curve was obtained by placing the probe of the Pitman 235 Isotope localisation monitor over the medial aspect of the calf at the site of the soleal veins and connecting the monitor to a pen recorder. The probe was removed whenever the image intensifier was switched on to avoid damage to it from radiation. A mark on the patient's skin ensured that the probe could be replaced exactly at the same position.

Selection of patients: The simultaneous clearance times of both sodium diatrizoate and ^{125}I-fibrinogen from the soleal and tibial veins have been determined in eight male volunteers with normal lower limbs prior to inguinal herniorrhaphy.

4. CLEARANCE OF ^{125}I-FIBRINOGEN FROM SOLEAL AND TIBIAL VEINS JUST BEFORE AND DURING OPERATION

Method: Thirty ml of normal saline containing 10 μCi of ^{125}I-fibrinogen were injected in a vein on the dorsum of the foot and directed into the tibial and soleal veins using the same technique described above. The mid-thigh cuff was then released and a clearance curve was obtained. This was performed just before the patients were anaesthetised and 20 minutes after the induction of anaesthesia while the operation was in progress.

Selection of patients: The clearance times of ^{125}I-fibrinogen from the soleal and tibial veins has been determined just before and during operation in 8 patients who had clinically normal legs.

5. OPTIMUM ELECTRIC STIMULATION OF CALF MUSCLES TO PREVENT STASIS

This part of the study was concerned with determining the most effective form of electric stimulation of the calf muscles to prevent stasis in the soleal veins.

Method: A doppler blood flow detector (Doptone) was placed at a constant angle and fixed to the skin over the femoral vein in the groin. A continuous recording of mean blood velocity was obtained via a pen recorder. The response of this instrument has been shown to be linear (Nicolaides, 1971d; Sampson *et al.*, 1970) and although the measurement of blood velocity in absolute units is not possible, changes in the mean velocity can be measured with an accuracy greater than 90 per cent. It was thus possible to record changes in the mean blood velocity of the femoral vein as a result of each calf muscle contraction while square wave electric stimuli of different intensity and duration with different resting periods between them were applied to the calf muscles. The electrodes were applied to the upper and lower part of the gastrocnemius muscle. They were covered by 4 layers of lint impregnated in normal saline.

Selection of patients: Ten consecutive patients have been studied during operation. The operating table and the patient's legs were kept horizontal.

6. EFFECT OF OPTIMUM PRE-OPERATIVE ELECTRIC STIMULATION OF CALF MUSCLES IN PREVENTING DEEP VEIN THROMBOSIS

In this final part of the study the optimum electric calf stimulus, as determined in part 5, was used in a clinical trial in an attempt to assess its effectiveness in preventing deep vein thrombosis.

Method: The patients were randomly divided into two groups. In the control group nothing specific was done to prevent deep vein thrombosis other than the usual hospital routine of prophylaxis. In the test group, as soon as the patient was anaesthetised two padded electrodes (6 × 15 cm) were applied to the upper and lower part of the posterior aspect of one calf, the right if the patient was born in an even year and left if born in an odd year. A 50 millisecond square wave current was applied every 5 seconds. The stimulating current was provided by a mains operated 'thrombophylactor' built by Stanley Cox Medical Equipment Division of Rank Precision Industries Ltd. according to the above specifications.

The intensity was always adjusted to produce a brisk plantar flexion of the foot without violent movement of the leg. This was discontinued at the end of the operation just before the patient would wake up.

All the patients were screened with the ^{125}I-fibrinogen test (Kakkar *et al.*, 1970). The thyroid gland was first blocked with sodium iodide (100 mg) and the ^{125}I-fibrinogen was given intravenously before operation. The legs were scanned before, immediately after operation, on the first and then on alternate days up to the 10th postoperative day. Using the Pitman 235 Isotape localisation monitor, the radioactivity at the various positions on the legs was exposed as a percentage of the heart count. A thrombus was diagnosed if there was a rise of 20 or more in the percentage value of radioactivity at the same position on two different days which persisted for more than 24 hours.

Selection of patients: A total of 116 patients over the age of 40 undergoing major surgical operations has been studied. Patients undergoing minor operations or operations on the legs or thyroid have been excluded. Patients placed in the lithotomy position also have been excluded. They were randomly divided into two groups. Fifty-six of them acted as controls, while the remaining sixty had calf muscles of one leg electrically stimulated during operation, the other leg also acting as a control.

RESULTS

1. SITE OF ORIGIN OF DEEP VEIN THROMBI

Thrombi were demonstrated by venography in only 70 (58 per cent) out of 121 patients with clinically suspected deep vein thrombosis. The remaining 51 (42 per cent) had a completely normal deep venous system (Table 7.1).

TABLE 7.1

121 PATIENTS WITH CLINICALLY SUSPECTED DEEP VENOUS THROMBOSIS

	D.V.T. on venography	*No D.V.T. on venography*
Soleal veins demonstrated	67 (68 venograms)	51 (63 venograms)
Soleal veins failed to be demonstrated	3	0
TOTALS	70 (58%)	51 (42%)

Bilateral venograms were performed in 13 patients.

The soleal veins (Fig. 7.1) were demonstrated in all patients investigated except three. These three patients had massive oedema with very tense limbs and little contrast medium could be made to enter the deep veins of the calf. There were thus 67 patients (68 venograms) in which both thrombi and soleal veins were demon-

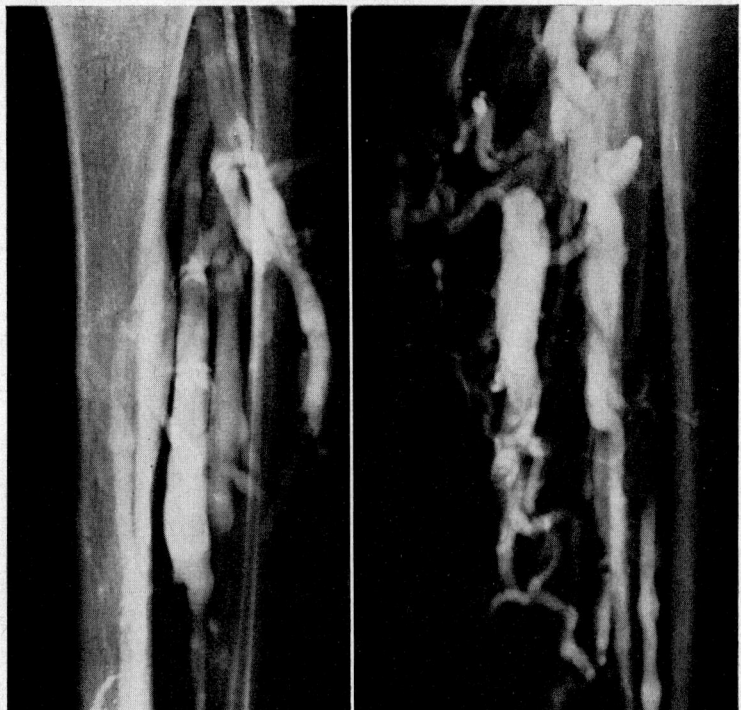

FIG. 7.1   FIG. 7.2

FIGS. 7.1 and 7.2. The soleal and tibial veins.

TABLE 7.2

DISTRIBUTION AND EXTENT OF THROMBI IN 68 VENOGRAMS

Vein involved	Degree of involvement in thrombotic process						
I.V.C.	—	—	—	—	—	—	—
Common iliac	—	—	—	—	—	+	+
Ext. iliac	—	—	—	—	+	+	+
Femoral	—	—	—	+	+	+	—
Popliteal	—	—	+	+	+	+*	—
Tibial	—	+	+	+	+	+	—
Soleal	+	+	+	+	+	+	—
No. of venograms	14	26	8	9	4	5	2

+ = Presence of thrombi
— = Normal vein
* = In two patients this segment was normal

strated. The distribution and extent of thrombi in these venograms is shown in Table 7.2.

In 14 limbs the thrombi were confined to the soleal veins (Fig. 7.3). In 26 limbs thrombi were present in the soleal and tibial veins (Fig. 7.4). In half of these patients the thrombi in the soleal veins

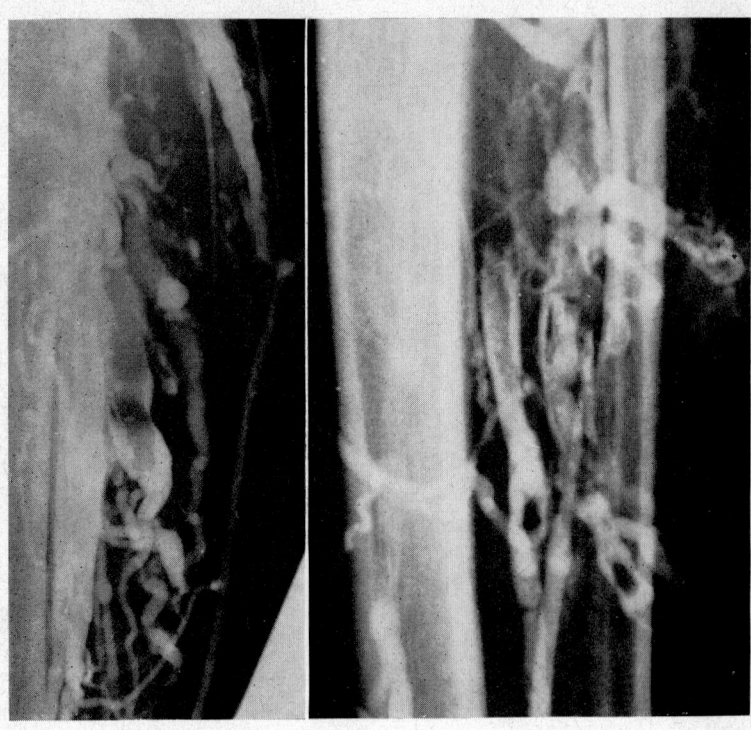

Fig. 7.3   Fig. 7.4

Fig. 7.3. Thrombi confined to the soleal veins.

Fig. 7.4. Thrombi in the soleal and tibial veins.

were actually seen to be in continuity with the thrombi in the tibial veins (Fig. 7.4). In eight limbs they were present in the soleal, tibial, and popliteal veins. In four limbs thrombi were present in the soleal, tibial, popliteal, femoral and external iliac veins. In five limbs thrombi were present in the soleal veins and in all the other deep veins right up to the common iliac vein, except that in two limbs the popliteal did not contain any thrombus (Table 7.2).

There were two limbs with occlusion of the external iliac vein only and with a normal venous system distally. One of these patients had Hodgkin's disease with massive glands in the pelvis and the other had retroperitoneal fibrosis. With the exception of these two cases, whenever there was a thrombus in the more proximal veins, there were also thrombi in the soleal and intervening veins.

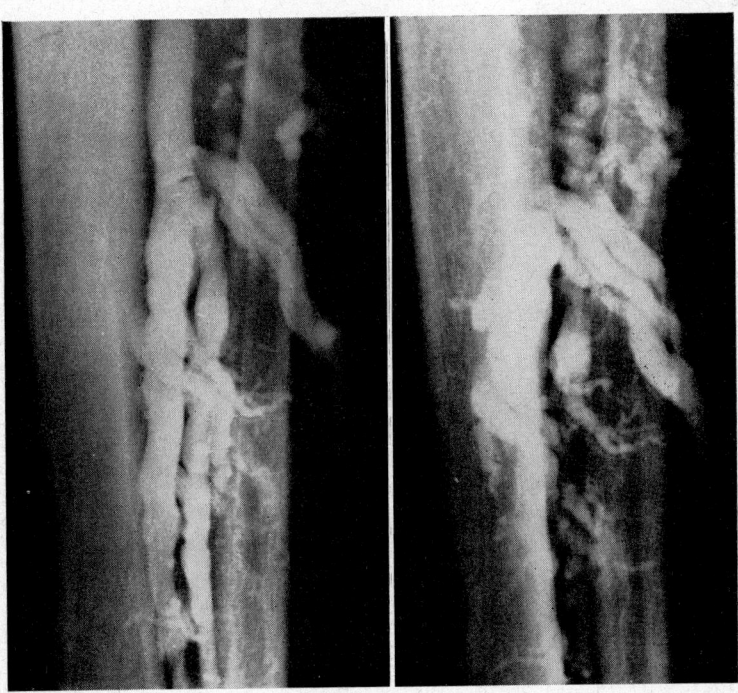

FIG. 7.5   FIG. 7.6

FIGS. 7.5 and 7.6. Contrast medium persisting in the soleal veins. The same leg before (Fig. 7.5) and after (Fig. 7.6) releasing the mid-thigh cuff.

2. CLEARANCE OF SODIUM DIATRIZOATE FROM TIBIAL AND SOLEAL VEINS

This was measured in six groups of patients.

Group I: Leg horizontal. In 16 patients, whose leg was kept horizontal when the mid-thigh cuff was released, the contrast medium disappeared first from the tibial veins, while it remained in the soleal veins for much longer (Figs. 7.5 and 7.6). The mean clearance time of contrast medium from the tibial veins was 1·1 minutes and from the soleal veins 9·6 minutes (Fig. 7.7). There was no correlation between age and the clearance times from the soleal veins (Fig. 7.8).

Group II: Leg horizontal with full length elastic stocking on. In five patients who had a full length elastic stocking on, the leg was also

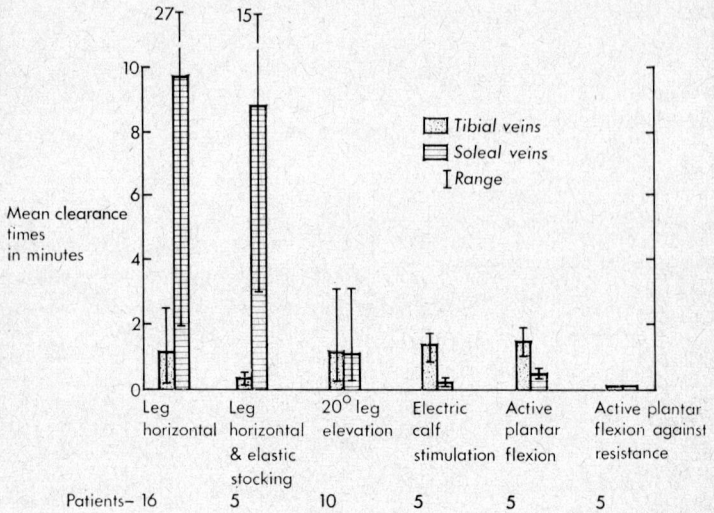

FIG. 7.7. Clearance of sodium diatrizoate from the tibial and soleal veins.

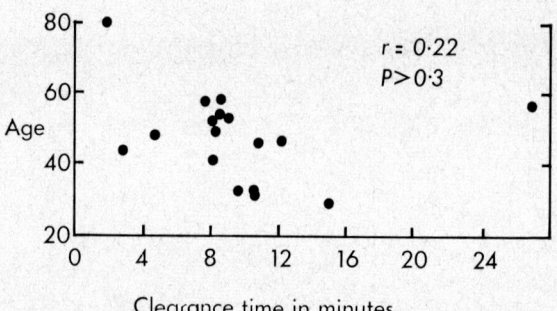

FIG. 7.8. Clearance rate related to age.

kept horizontal. The clearance from the soleal veins was similar to Group I, but there was a tendency for the tibial veins to empty faster (Fig. 7.7).

Group III: 20° leg elevation. In ten patients whose leg was elevated 20°, the tibial and soleal veins emptied simultaneously. The mean clearance time for the tibial veins was 1·0 minutes and for the soleal veins 1·1 minutes.

Group IV: Active plantar flexion of the foot. Five patients were asked to plantar-flex the foot once every four seconds after the mid-thigh cuff was released while keeping the leg horizontal. The contrast medium disappeared from the soleal veins first within 0·5 minutes and from the tibial veins within 1·4 minutes.

Group V: Electric calf stimulation. In five patients the calf muscles were stimulated by electrodes (faradic) to contract and produce a powerful but tolerable plantar flexion of the foot every four seconds after the mid-thigh cuff was removed. The contrast medium disappeared from the soleal veins first within 0·2 minutes and from the tibial veins within 1·45 minutes.

Group VI: Plantar flexion of the foot against resistance. Five patients were asked to plantar flex the foot against resistance after the mid-thigh cuff was released. In these patients two plantar flexions were enough to empty both the soleal and tibial veins of contrast medium. The fluoroscopic changes in groups IV, V, and VI have been recorded on cine.

3. SIMULTANEOUS CLEARANCE OF SODIUM DIATRIZOATE AND ^{125}I-FIBRINOGEN FROM TIBIAL AND SOLEAL VEINS

The clearance curves obtained were biphasic in all eight patients investigated (Fig. 7.9). By intermittently screening and observing the clearance of sodium diatrizoate on the image intensifier it was noted that the disappearance of the contrast medium from the tibial veins coincided with the end of phase I and from the soleal

TABLE 7.3

SIMULTANEOUS CLEARANCE OF HYPAQUE AND ^{125}I-FIBRINOGEN IN EIGHT PATIENTS

	Clearance time of hypaque (mins)		*Clearance time of ^{125}I-fibrinogen (mins)*	
	Tibial veins	*Soleal veins*	*Tibial veins*	*Soleal veins*
1.	3·3	9·6	3·7	10·0
2.	0·5	2·6	0·5	2·7
3.	0·8	2·4	0·8	2·4
4.	0·5	5·5	0·5	5·4
5.	1·2	5·2	1·0	5·0
6.	1·5	7·3	1·5	7·3
7.	0·7	3·5	0·9	3·7
8.	1·4	6·3	1·4	6·5

veins with the end of phase II (Fig. 7.9). The final endpoint was the point on the clearance curve after which the fall in radioactivity was less than 2 per cent of the initial count per minute. The final level of radioactivity was the same in both legs.

The mean clearance times obtained by the fluoroscopic method were in agreement with the clearance times obtained by the isotopic method (Table 7.3).

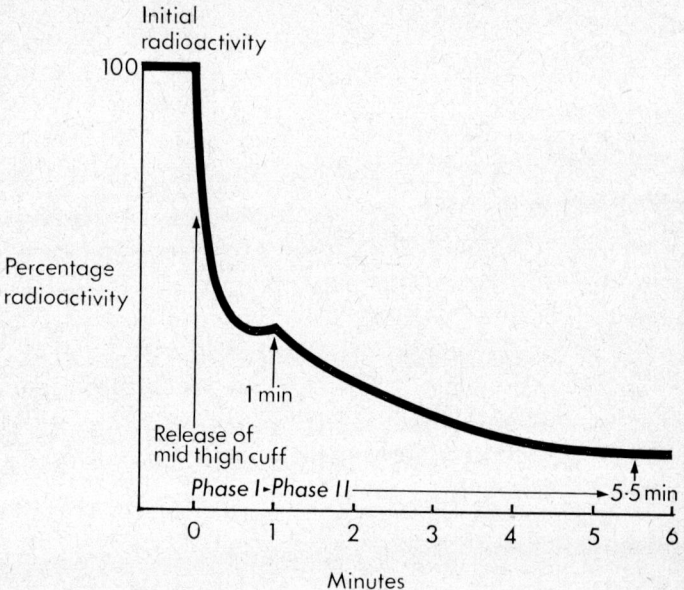

FIG. 7.9. Clearance curve of ^{125}I-fibrinogen from the tibial and soleal veins.

4. CLEARANCE OF ^{125}I-FIBRINOGEN BEFORE AND DURING OPERATION

The mean clearance times of ^{125}I-fibrinogen from the tibial and soleal veins before and during operation are shown in Fig. 7.10. The mean clearance time of the ^{125}I-fibrinogen from the tibial veins was essentially the same before and during operation, but the mean clearance time from the soleal veins was twice as long during operation.

5. OPTIMUM ELECTRIC STIMULATION OF CALF MUSCLES TO PREVENT STASIS

There was a brief but marked increase of the mean velocity of blood in the femoral vein with every calf contraction. Fluoroscopic and cine phlebographic studies in Part 2 of this investigation (see Group IV) have already demonstrated that each calf muscle contraction forces proximally a large volume of blood (stroke volume) which comes out of the soleal and tibial veins. It is reasonable to assume that the greater stroke volume will be produced by the stimulus which will also produce the greatest increase in the femoral vein velocity.

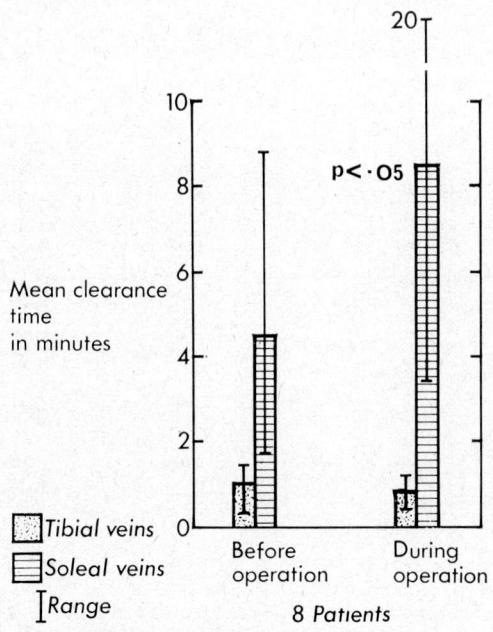

FIG. 7.10. Clearance of ^{125}I-fibrinogen from tibial and soleal veins in the same patients before and during operation.

The most appropriate intensity/duration combination was that which produced a brisk plantar flexion of the foot without violent movement of the leg. More powerful stimuli produced violent leg movements and only a small additional increase in the femoral vein velocity. A resting period of less than 4 seconds did not allow the soleal veins to fill completely before the next stimulus and this resulted in a progressive reduction in femoral vein velocity. A resting period of more than 5 seconds allowed the soleal veins to fill during the resting period so that successive stimuli resulted in the same maximum femoral vein velocity.

6. EFFECT OF OPTIMUM ELECTRIC STIMULATION OF CALF MUSCLES IN PREVENTING DEEP VEIN THROMBOSIS

In the control group, 18 (23 per cent) out of 56 patients developed deep vein thrombosis. In 7 patients the thrombi were bilateral. There were thus 25 limbs with deep vein thrombosis; 13 right and 12 left. All thrombi has started in the calf. Two extended into the popliteal and one into the femoral vein. The time the thrombi formed is shown in Fig. 7.11.

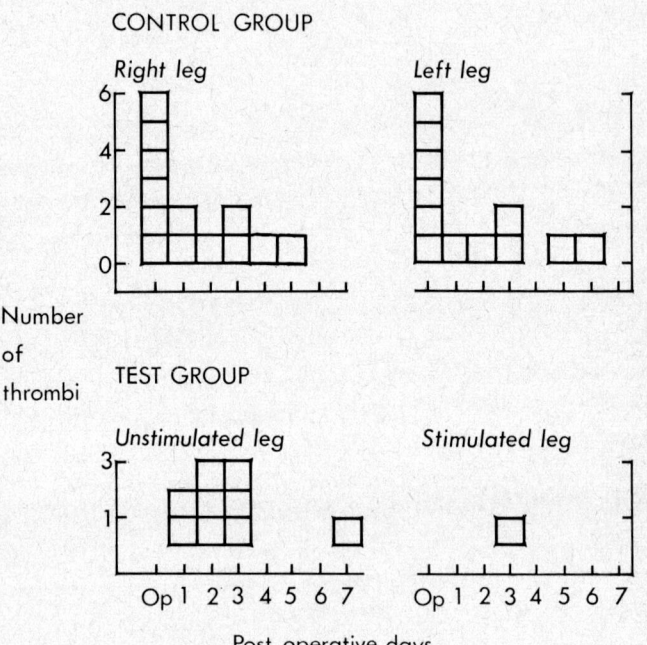

FIG. 7.11. Effect of electrical stimulation of the calf muscles on the incidence of deep vein thrombosis.

In the group of patients who had calf stimulation on one leg during operation, 9 (15 per cent) out of 60 patients developed deep vein thrombosis. In only one patient were the thrombi bilateral. In the remaining eight the thrombi occurred in the unstimulated leg. The time they formed is also shown in Fig. 7.11.

In the test group of patients, using the unstimulated leg as control in a sequential analysis with $2\alpha = 0.5$, $1 - \beta = 0.95$, $\theta_1 = 0.85$ (probability of 5 per cent), the trial favours calf stimulation (Fig. 7.12).

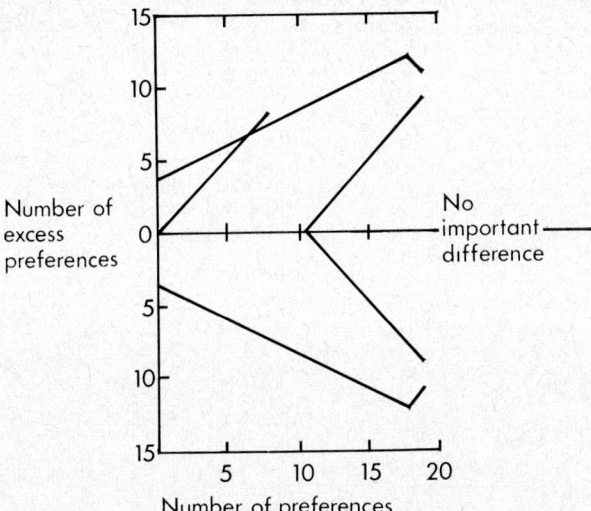

FIG. 7.12. Sequential analysis of the effect of electrical stimulation of the calf muscles.

If the incidence of deep vein thrombosis in the stimulated leg in the test group is compared with either the right or left leg of the control group, the difference is also significant (Fisher's exact test: $p = 0.00028$; Table 7.4).

It is interesting to note that in the test group the incidence of deep vein thrombosis in the unstimulated leg (15 per cent) is less than in

TABLE 7.4
RESULTS OF CALF STIMULATION TRIAL

		No D.V.T.	D.V.T.	Total	Fisher's exact test
Control Group	R. Leg	43	13 (23%)	56	
	L. Leg	44	12 (21%)	56	
Test Group	Stimulated Leg	59	1 (1.6%)	60	$p = 0.00028$
	Unstimulated Leg	51	9 (15%)	60	$p = 0.10$

the control group. Although this is not significant (Table 7.4), Fig. 7.11 shows that this is due to the absence of any thrombi occurring during the operation. If this is compared with the relatively high incidence of deep vein thrombosis on the day of operation in the control group (Table 7.5) this is significant (Fisher's exact test: $p = 0.011$).

TABLE 7.5

INCIDENCE OF THROMBI OCCURRING ON DAY OF OPERATION

		No D.V.T.	D.V.T.	Total
Control Group	R. Leg	50	6	56
	L. Leg	50	6	56
Test Group	Unstimulated Leg	60	0*	60

*Fisher's exact test: $p = 0.011$.

Finally, in order to show that the two groups of patients are truly comparable, the distribution of various factors known to predispose to deep vein thrombosis in the patients studied are shown in Table 7.6.

TABLE 7.6

DISTRIBUTION OF FACTORS FAVOURING D.V.T.

	Mean age	Obesity	History of DVT	History of PE	Varicose veins	Malignancy
Control Group	56 ± 12.4	12	3	1	7	14
Test Group	52 ± 13.8	16	3	2	5	11

None of the patients in this trial had any complications as a result of the methods of investigation described.

DISCUSSION

There has been considerable controversy about the origin of thrombi in the deep veins of the legs. Some authors believe that a considerable proportion of thrombi start in the proximal large veins of the leg and pelvis (McLachlin and Paterson, 1951; Sevitt and Gallagher, 1961) while others believe that the great majority of thrombi start in the veins of the lower leg (Bauer, 1940; Bauer, 1964; Dodd and Cockett, 1956; Gibbs, 1957). It has been suspected for some time that the soleal veins are important as a site of thrombosis (Cotton and Clarke, 1965). Information on the site of origin of thrombi is of importance because any attempt at prophylaxis would have to take into account where the thrombus commences, whether it is related to stasis, and if so, how stasis can be prevented.

The results of the first part of this study (Table 7.2) show that, in some patients, thrombi have been confined to the soleal veins. It has also been shown that with a few exceptions, whenever there are thrombi proximally, there are always thrombi present in the soleal and intervening veins. It can be argued that the presence of soleal thrombi, whenever there is proximal thrombosis, may be due to peripheral extension of thrombi arising in the more proximal veins. This, however, does not happen as shown by studies using the ^{125}I-fibrinogen test in surgical (Flanc et al., 1968; Negus et al., 1968) gynaecological (Friend, 1971), orthopaedic (Field et al., 1971), urological (Nicolaides et al., 1972), obstetric (Friend, 1970) and medical patients (Murray et al., 1970; Nicolaides et al., 1971a). These studies have in fact shown that thrombi practically always start in the calf and extend proximally. If this evidence is taken in conjunction with the distribution of the thrombi found in the present study, then the only possible conclusion is that, in the majority of patients, venous thrombi start in the soleal veins.

Previous studies have suggested that stasis occurs in the soleal veins and that this is particularly so in older patients (McLachlin et al., 1960). The results of the present clearance studies of sodium diatrizoate confirm that there is considerable stasis in the soleal veins when the leg is horizontal, but this is not related to age (Fig. 7.8). This means that the higher incidence of deep vein thrombosis associated with elderly patients may be related to factors other than stasis.

Elastic stockings had some effect on hastening the clearance of contrast medium from the tibial veins, but had no effect on the rate of emptying of the soleal veins. These results would be compatible with the work of Makin and his colleagues (1969) who showed that 'Tubigrip' increases the velocity of venous return in the legs and would also explain why elastic stockings had no effect on the incidence of deep vein thrombosis (Rosengarten et al., 1970). Stasis in the soleal veins, however, was prevented by 20° leg elevation, active plantar flexion of the foot and electric calf stimulation. It appears that active plantar flexion is more effective than leg elevation in preventing stasis in the soleal veins. The best way to prevent stasis in the soleal veins is active plantar flexion against resistance in the conscious patient, and electric calf muscle stimulation in the unconscious patient.

By measuring the simultaneous clearance of sodium diatrizoate and ^{125}I-fibrinogen from the veins of the calf it has been shown that the clearance of the protein-bound isotope directed into the deep veins is an accurate method of assessing stasis without fluoroscopy. Using this technique it has been demonstrated that stasis in the soleal veins is markedly increased during operation.

Of the methods studied electric calf stimulation appears to be the most suitable and most effective in preventing stasis during operation. Calf stimulation during operation had been shown to reduce the incidence of deep vein thrombosis (Browse and Negus, 1970) but this had not been confirmed by subsequent studies (De Jode et al., 1970). It may well be that the difference in the results is due to different stimuli used.

Cine-phlebographic studies have shown that the soleus muscle and its veins act as a peripheral pump (Almen and Nylander, 1962) filling during relaxation and emptying during contraction. The optimum electric calf stimulus is defined as that which produces the maximum output from the calf (stroke volume) which can be maintained during the operation. This can only be maintained if the stimulus is applied at a rate not more frequent than 15 per minute. Stimuli more frequent than this produce a progressive fall in the stroke volume because the short interval between them does not allow complete filling of the soleal veins.

The stimulus used in the final part of the present investigation has proved quite effective, producing a 92 per cent reduction in the incidence of deep vein thrombosis in the stimulated leg. It has also prevented the formation of thrombi in the unstimulated leg during operation. These findings pose two questions: (1) Why electric calf stimulation during the operation has prevented thrombi forming during the post-operative period? (2) Why has it prevented thrombi forming in the opposite leg during the operation?

Only a hypothesis can be suggested at his stage. In answer to the first question it may be suggested that perhaps a lot more thrombi than previously suspected start during the operation and are now prevented. At this stage they might be too small to be detected even with the ^{125}I-fibrinogen test. In answer to the second question it may be that the muscular contractions release fibrinolytic activator in the blood which acts not only locally but also systemically. There is good evidence that muscle activity increases the fibrinolytic activity in the blood (Fearnley, 1965) and that muscles are a source of plasminogen activators to the circulation (Menon, 1969). It has also been shown that the same occurs in patients having E.C.T. without relaxants, but not if muscle relaxants are administered prior to E.C.T. (Worowski et al., 1970).

The results of this trial, which demonstrate that electric calf stimulation during operation can prevent deep vein thrombosis in the stimulated leg, suggest that if both legs were stimulated this would practically abolish deep vein thrombosis. This would be easy with the 'thrombophylactor' since it has the facility for stimulating both legs. It should however be pointed out that, although this method is simple and safe, it has its limitations. It cannot be used in patients in the lithotomy position or in orthopaedic patients. It may well be that simple methods that prevent hypercoagulability (Kakkar et al., 1971) may prove more practical in these patients (Nicolaides, 1972).

REFERENCES

ALMEN, T. and NYLANDER, G. (1962) *Acta Radiol.*, **57,** 264.
ATKINS, P. and HAWKINS, L. A. (1965) *Lancet*, **2,** 1217.
BAUER, G. (1940) *Acta Chir. Scand.*, Suppl. 61, **84,** 1.
BAUER, G. (1964) *Amer. J. Cardiol.*, **14,** 29.
BROWSE, N. L. and NEGUS, D. (1970) *Brit. med. J.*, **3,** 615.
COTTON, L. T. and CLARKE, C. (1965) *Annals. R. Coll. Surg. Eng.* **36,** 214.
DODD, H. and COCKETT, F. B. (1956) *The Pathology and Surgery of the Veins of the Lower Limb*. Edinburgh and London: Livingstone.
FEARNLEY, G. S. (1965) *Fibrinolysis*. London: Arnold.
FIELD, E. S. et al. (1971) *Brit. J. Surg.*, **58,** 873.
FLANC, C. et al. (1968) *Brit. J. Surg.*, **55,** 742.
FLANC, C. et al. (1969) *Lancet*, **1,** 478.
FRIEND, J. R. and KAKKAR, V.V. (1970) *J. Obstet. Gynaec. Brit. Cwlth.*, **77,** 820.
FRIEND, J. R. (1971) Personal communication.
GIBBS, N. M. (1957), *Brit. J. Surg.* **45,** 209.
HILLS, N. H. et al. (1971) *Brit. J. Surg.*, **58,** 855.
DE JODE, L. R. J. et al. (1970) *Brit. med. J.*, **3,** 56.
KAKKAR, V. V. et al. (1969) *Lancet*, **2,** 230.
KAKKAR, V. V. et al. (1970) *Lancet*, **1,** 540.
KAKKAR, V. V. et al. (1971) *Lancet*, **2,** 669.
MCLACHLIN, J. and PATERSON, J. C. (1951) *Surgery, Gyn. and Obstet.*, **93,** 8.
MCLACHLIN, A. D. et al. (1960) *Ann. Surg.*, **152,** 678.
MAKIN, G. S. et al. (1969) *Brit. J. Surg.*, **56,** 369.
MENON, S. (1969) *J. Assoc. Phys. Ind.*, **17,** 141.
MURRAY, T. S. et al. (1970) *Lancet*, **2,** 792.
NEGUS, D. et al. (1968) *Brit. J. Surg.* **55,** 835.
NICOLAIDES, A. N. et al. (1971a) *Brit. med. J.* **1,** 432.
NICOLAIDES, A. N. et al. (1971b) *Brit. J. Surg.* **58,** 307.
NICOLAIDES, A. N. et al. (1971c) *Brit. J. Radiol.* **44,** 653.

NICOLAIDES, A. N. (1971d).
NICOLAIDES, A. N. (1972) *Modern Geriatrics*, **2,** April issue.
NICOLAIDES, A. N. et al. (1972) *Brit. J. Surg.*, in press.
PENICK, G. D. et al. (1965) *Fed. Proc.*, **24,** 835.
ROSENGARTEN, D. S. et al. (1970) *Brit. J. Surg.*, **57,** 296.
ROSENGARTEN, D. S. and LAIRD, J. (1971) *Brit. J. Surg.*, **58,** 182.
SABRI, S. et al. (1971) *Brit. med. J.* **3,** 82.
SAMPSON, D. et al. (1970) *Brit. med. J.*, **1,** 340.
SEVITT, S. and GALLAGHER, N. (1961) *Brit. J. Surg.*, **48,** 475.
DE WEESE, J. A. and ROGOFF, S. M. (1963) *Surgery*, **53,** 99.
WESSLER, S. and YIN, E. T. (1968) *Prog. Hemat.*, **6,** 201.
WOROWSKI, K. et al. (1970) *Coagulation*, **3,** 23.

8 Diagnosis of Deep Venous Thrombosis and its Sequelae by Doppler Ultrasound Detection

B. Sigel, W. R. Felix, Jr., J. Ipsen and
G. L. Popky

The diagnosis of lower limb deep venous thrombosis by clinical examination alone is unreliable. This has led to a search for other diagnostic procedures which provide more valid information about the tendency to thrombosis, the evolution of thrombosis, or the presence of established thrombi in the deep veins of the lower limbs. We have developed a Doppler ultrasound technique for the detection of deep venous occlusion due to thrombosis and the assessment of valve competency in the post-phlebitic state. The purpose of this paper is briefly to describe the method, present its capabilities and limitations, and indicate how we have applied it clinically.

DESCRIPTION OF METHOD

The instrumentation has been described and we have published previously a detailed account of the technique which we use to diagnose deep vein occlusion and incompetence of valves (Sigel et al., 1968). Consequently, only a brief summary of our technique will be presented here.

The Doppler ultrasound blood velocity detector senses blood flow by the shift in frequency produced by the backscatter of high frequency sound from moving red cells. We have used mostly a continuous wave Doppler ultrasound detector of 5 megaHertz frequency. The 10 megaHertz instrument may be used also for this purpose. A number of battery operated portable detectors is now available commercially in the United States and Europe.

Because ultrasound does not travel well through a gaseous

*Supported by grants from the National Heart Institute (Public Health Service) No. HE-11774, the John A. Hartford Foundation, and by Part I Research Funds of the Veterans Administration.

medium, an acoustical coupling gel is applied between the transducer and the skin. The transducer is composed of two ceramic crystals set adjacent and usually at a slight angle to each other. One crystal transmits the sound and the other receives the backscattered signal. The difference in frequency between the transmitted and received signal produced by the Doppler shift indicates the velocity of the target particles (red cells). Thus, with a fast flowing stream, the Doppler shift is greater than with a slow flowing stream. As used transcutaneously, this device cannot accurately measure flow velocity because the angle between the transducer and the blood vessel cannot be known precisely. However, it is very suitable as a sensor of flow.

Most instruments include a filter to remove the lower frequency noise. While this greatly facilitates detection of flow in rapid streams and is ideal for arteries, flow in slower moving streams may not be detectable. The Doppler shifted frequency difference between transmitted and received signals may be provided as audio signals which can be heard readily by earphones or loud-speaker. These signals also may be displayed by a sound spectrum analyser or, upon signal modification, as a simple analogue curve on a chart recorder. In our work, we rely almost exclusively on the audible signal.

Since most commercial Doppler ultrasound detectors will not detect a relatively slow velocity (e.g. below 6 cm/sec), the absence of a signal from a vessel does not necessarily mean 'no flow'. It can also mean 'slow flow', which may be quite normal in veins. To overcome this limitation, we have manually compressed the extremity to produce a pulse wave or augmentation flow wave which propagates up and down the deep venous system at greater velocity than the flow of blood in veins. Propagation of this wave distally is damped by normally functioning valves. Propagation centrally may be ultrasonically detected as far as one metre or more proximal to the site of compression. This pulse wave produces a transient augmented flow signal which we have termed Augmented or A sound. This A sound may be superimposed on a spontaneous flow signal or S sound which is cyclical with respiration. Fig. 8.1 is a sound spectrogram of an A sound obtained from a vein.

Our approach to diagnosing venous disease is based almost entirely on the use of augmented flow signals or A sounds as heard through a loudspeaker. The examiner must judge whether the A sound is present, diminished, or absent. S sounds are also judged in terms of their pitch and cyclical occurrence in phase with respiration. S sounds which are high-pitched and continuous (not cyclical) indicate rapid venous flow as in a collateral channel and are sometimes helpful in indirectly suggesting occlusion.

The Doppler ultrasound examination as we use it is an integral part of the clinical examination for venous disease. We first inspect and palpate the lower extremities. Then we employ the ultrasound detector as we use the stethoscope in the examination of the chest or abdomen. The ultrasound examination may be complete or partial depending on whether we are interested in detecting occlusion and incompetent valves or occlusion alone. Usually we perform initially a complete examination. Subsequently, if re-examination is desired within a few days of the first examination, we perform only a partial examination to determine the occurrence of venous thrombosis in the intervening period.

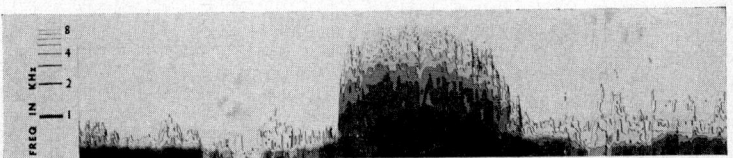

Fig. 8.1. Sound spectrogram of an augmented flow signal or A sound which is superimposed on the spontaneous flow signal or S sound. The frequency of the Doppler shift is represented on the ordinate and the time represented on the abscissa is about 4.5 seconds. The intensity (amplitude) is depicted in the contour plot with the darkest area representing the greatest amount of energy. The S sounds are at either end of the spectrogram and the A sound in the centre. The peak frequency of the S sound is generally below 1 KHz while that of the A sound ranges between 4 and 8 KHz.

COMPLETE EXAMINATION OF DEEP VENOUS SYSTEM FOR OCCLUSION AND INCOMPETENT VALVES

Complete examination of the lower limb for both occlusion and incompetent valves comprises ultrasound examination performed at three locations: (1) common femoral vein: (2) posterior tibial vein; and (3) popliteal vein. The examination is performed with the patient supine in bed or on an examining table. The head of the bed should be slightly elevated to maintain a larger pool of venous blood in the lower extremities. Most of our examinations are now performed by a nurse or by technicians.

The common femoral vein at the inguinal ligament is examined first. The transducer is applied over the vein just medial to the femoral artery pulse. An S sound is usually present in phase with the patient's respiration. The lower thigh is compressed manually and the examiner notes the occurrence of the A sound (Fig. 8.2). With the position of the transducer maintained, the calf is compressed and the presence of the A sound ascertained. The process is repeated with passive dorsiflexion of the foot.

The posterior tibial vein is examined next behind the medial malleolus. S sounds which are usually present at the femoral vein are in most instances absent at the posterior tibial vein. The calf at the junction of the mid and lower third is compressed and the presence of an A sound determined. Following release, the examiner again notes the presence of an A sound. With the transducer position steady, the procedure is repeated distal to the transducer with compression and release of the foot.

The femoral and posterior tibial veins are examined in the opposite extremity and the patient is asked to turn to a prone position for

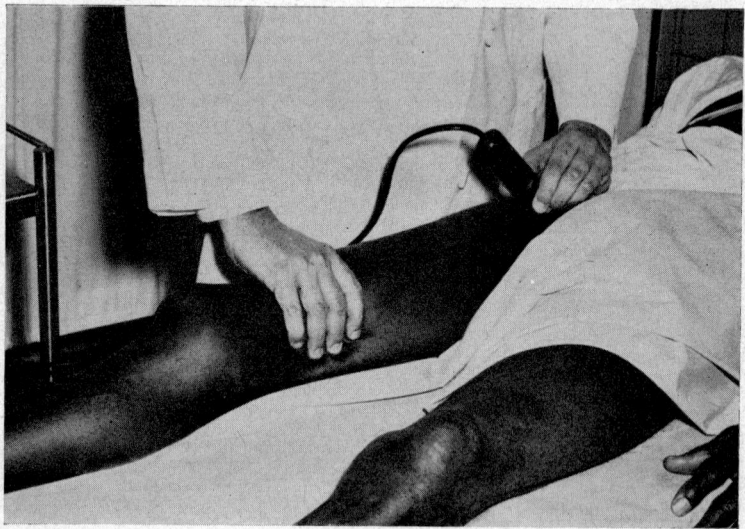

FIG. 8.2. Elicitation of distal positive femoral A sound by lower thigh compression.

examination of the popliteal veins. To facilitate examination of the popliteal vein, a pillow or other prop is placed beneath the leg to permit 10–15° flexion of the knee. We have found that full hyperextension of the leg can obliterate the S sound in the popliteal flow suggesting a functional interference to flow. The popliteal vein signal is either with or lateral to the artery signal. Often it is not possible to separate the artery from the vein signal. S sounds are detected in about half of the examinations. The lower calf is compressed and released and the presence of A sounds noted. Compression proximal to the transducer is conducted at three locations: lower third, middle third, and upper third of the thigh.

PARTIAL EXAMINATION OF DEEP VENOUS SYSTEM FOR OCCLUSION

For determining the presence of occlusion only, the examination may be limited to the common femoral vein sites with compression of the thigh, leg and dorsiflexion of the foot. This shortens examination time by an experienced observer to 5 to 6 minutes and obviates having the patient turned. The examination of the femoral vein is conducted in all respects similar to that in the complete examination.

INTERPRETATION OF DOPPLER ULTRASOUND EXAMINATION

For descriptive purposes, we have designated A sounds according to site of compression and whether they have been produced by the actual compression or release of compression. Thus, we term A sounds produced by compressing beyond the transducer as distal A sounds and those produced by compression central to the transducer as proximal A sounds. A sounds produced by the actual compression are termed positive and those produced by release of compression are termed negative.

ULTRASOUND DIAGNOSIS OF OCCLUSION

The Doppler ultrasound diagnosis of occlusion is made by the absence or marked diminution of the distal positive femoral A sound. If the distal positive femoral A sound from lower thigh compression is normal but absent or reduced from calf compression, we interpret the examination as revealing leg vein occlusion. If the distal positive A sound from thigh compression is also abnormal, our ultrasound diagnosis becomes femoral vein occlusion. We grade the extent of occlusion as partial if diminished distal positive femoral A sounds are obtained or as complete if the distal positive femoral A sounds are absent.

Diminution or absence of distal positive popliteal A sounds also indicates leg vein occlusion. However, in our experience, the distal positive femoral A sound is a more reliable sign. The absence of proximal negative A sounds will also indicate occlusion but duplicates what can be learned from the distal positive A sound. We no longer use these signs and base our examination for occlusion entirely upon the distal positive femoral A sound.

ULTRASOUND DIAGNOSIS OF INCOMPETENCE OF VALVES

Incompetence of valves is determined by the occurrence of two types of A sound which normally should not be present. Distal negative A sounds from release of thigh compression, calf compressions, or foot compression denotes incompetence in the valves of the femoral, leg and foot veins respectively. Proximal positive popliteal A sounds produced by compressing the mid and upper thirds of the thigh indicate incompetence of the femoral vein valves. The presence of proximal positive posterior tibial A sounds is probably the best ultrasound method, in our hands, for diagnosis of the post-phlebitic syndrome involving the deep veins of the leg.

CAPABILITIES AND LIMITATIONS OF DOPPLER ULTRASOUND DETECTION

Prior to utilizing the Doppler ultrasound technique on a wide scale in epidemiologic and clinical application, we performed a validative study to correlate the ultrasound method with phlebography or operative and autopsy findings and to compare it with clinical examination (Sigel et al., 1970). Among the first 500 patients examined by us, we obtained confirmation of findings by phlebography in 139 and by operation or autopsy in 8. In these 147 patients, information was available on 248 extremities because phlebograms were usually performed bilaterally. A number of patients examined by phlebography had negative findings on clinical and ultrasound examination but were suspected of having recent pulmonary embolism.

TABLE 8.1

SENSITIVITY OF ULTRASOUND AND CLINICAL EXAMINATION IN DETECTING OCCLUSION

	Ultrasound	*Clinical*
Number of extremities found occluded by validating procedure	83	83
Extremities correctly identified by examination as occluded	63	45
Sensitivity	75·9%	54·2%

The evaluation of a screening surveillance procedure is best expressed in terms of sensitivity and specificity compared to a more definitive final outcome (Thorner and Remein, 1961). Sensitivity is defined as the number of positive extremities obtained divided by the actual number of extremities proven to have venous occlusion by phlebography or anatomic confirmation. Specificity is defined as the number of negative extremities observed divided by the number of extremities proven to be nonoccluded. Sensitivity and specificity are usually multiplied by 100 to present these values as percentages. Comparison of Doppler ultrasound and clinical methods of validating examinations in the diagnosis of deep venous occlusion revealed that the ultrasound examination was significantly more sensitive and specific than clinical examinations (See Tables 8.1 and 8.2).

TABLE 8.2
SPECIFICITY OF ULTRASOUND AND CLINICAL EXAMINATION IN DETECTING OCCLUSION

	Ultrasound	Clinical
Number of extremities found non-occluded by validation	165	165
Extremities correctly identified by examination as negative for occlusion	150	106
Specificity	90·9%	64·2%

Comparison of Doppler ultrasound and clinical methods was also compared to phlebography in the diagnosis of incompetent deep venous valves. The ultrasound examination was more sensitive but less specific than clinical examination (See Tables 8.3 and 8.4).

TABLE 8.3
SENSITIVITY OF ULTRASOUND AND CLINCIAL EXAMINATION FOR INCOMPETENCE OF DEEP VENOUS VALVES

	Ultrasound	Clinical
Number of extremities with demonstrated abnormal valves by phlebography	72	72
Extremities correctly identified by examination as containing incompetent deep venous valves	55	38
Sensitivity	76·4%	52·8%

In order to quantitate better the limitation of the ultrasound method, we reassessed sensitivity in terms of the location of venous occlusion and the estimated duration of the venous thrombosis.

The sensitivity of the ultrasound technique in relation to the distribution of the thrombi within the deep veins was determined in the following manner. All confirmed thromboses were classified according to occlusion of the leg veins alone or occlusion of the femoral vein either alone or in combination with the leg veins. Of the 83 positive extremities, occlusion in leg veins only occurred in 28 extremities or about one-third of the instances. The sensitivity of the ultrasound examination was 60·7 per cent (17 of 28 extremities) in the extremities with leg vein occlusion alone. Where the femoral vein was occluded, the sensitivity was 83·6 per cent (46 of 55 extremities).

TABLE 8.4

SPECIFICITY OF ULTRASOUND AND CLINICAL EXAMINATION FOR INCOMPETENCE OF DEEP VENOUS VALVES

	Ultrasound	Clinical
Number of extremities with normal appearing valves or phlebograms	124	124
Extremities correctly identified as normal in terms of valve function	84	98
Specificity	67·7%	79·0%

The sensitivity of the ultrasound method according to the duration of the occluding process was estimated by reassessing the chronicity of venous occlusion in the phlebograms. Employing an arbitrary set of criteria for 'new' and 'old' occlusion as defined by the radiologist, we estimated the sensitivity of ultrasound diagnosis in detecting 'new' occlusion as 78·1 per cent and in detecting 'old' occlusion as 67·5 per cent.

CLINICAL APPLICATION

We have applied ultrasound and clinical examination of venous disease in two ways. First, we have been conducting a study of prevalence and incidence of venous disease in hopitalised surgical patients. Second, we have seen a number of patients in consultation. In all, we have performed about 8500 examinations in over 5000 patients. About 1800 of these patients were seen in consultation.

The epidemiologic study is still underway and the data from this is still preliminary. In the first 1900 patients examined, the prevalence of venous occlusion in patients coming to elective operation was 8·6 per cent in terms of positive clinical findings and 0·9 per cent in terms of positive ultrasound findings. The incidence of disease at seven days post-operatively was 11·8 per cent by clinical and 2·6 per cent by ultrasound criteria. At fourteen days, patients who were still in hospital had a 16·8 per cent incidence of occlusion by clinical and 3·4 per cent incidence by ultrasound signs.

We have been asked to see primarily two types of patients in consultation. The first type has been patients in whom pulmonary embolism has been suspected or confirmed by angiography. Ultrasound examination was sought to attempt to localise the site of thrombosis. Where the ultrasound examination has been positive, we have usually not performed phlebography. However, in instances of negative findings on the ultrasound examination, we have continued to employ phlebography where a more certain diagnosis is required to make decisions regarding management. The second group of patients presented with problems in the lower limbs. These have included patients with lower extremity pain, swelling or skin changes suggestive of the post-phlebitic syndrome, where a question regarding the presence of thrombosis existed. The ultrasound examination has been particularly helpful in differentiating between the oedema of venous thrombosis and that produced by congestive failure or cirrhosis.

DISCUSSION

The Doppler ultrasound method of diagnosing venous disease has strength and weakness which the clinician must bear in mind. The advantages of the procedure include the following: (1) superior sensitivity and specificity of diagnosis compared to clinical appraisal, particularly in involvement of the femoral vein; (2) safety because of the non-invasive nature of the technique; (3) ability to diagnose occlusion as high as the common femoral vein; (4) rapidity of performing the examination in a few minutes; (5) no appreciable delay between a decision to obtain the examination and the results of the test; (6) simplicity and economy in performing the examination; (7) acceptance by physicians and patients; (8) ability to perform examination in operated or traumatized extremities; and (9) ability to obtain information about the competency of deep venous valves. The limitations of the method are: (1) high false negative findings (almost 40 per cent) if the calf veins alone are involved; and (2) inability to detect thrombi in the pelvic veins.

The advantages of the method taken together indicate that this is a very suitable procedure for mass application in screening and surveillance, particularly for the detection of more extensive thrombosis involving the femoral vein. The procedure has less value in the diagnosis of early incipient thrombosis which has not produced a significant degree of obstruction.

A number of methods have been described in this symposium which are designed to provide information about the tendency to thrombosis, the evolution of thrombosis, and the presence of established thrombi in the deep veins of the lower extremities. It is difficult to assess the relative merit of each test because not only are different procedures being considered but also different stages in the course of the disease. It appears to us that the final resolution of this problem must await the determination of the value of each procedure and variable in predicting the occurrence of the complications of venous disease—namely, pulmonary embolism and the post-phlebitic syndrome. This we believe should be the ultimate standard of evaluation used by clinical investigators involved in the early detection of venous thrombosis.

SUMMARY

Thrombosis and valve incompetence in the deep venous system of the lower extremity may be detected by a Doppler ultrasound technique with much greater precision than clinical examination alone.

The advantages of the procedure are:
> Superior sensitivity and specificity of diagnosis compared to clinical appraisal, particularly in involvement of the femoral vein.
> Safety because of the non-invasive nature of the technique.
> Ability to diagnose occlusion as high as the common femoral vein.
> Rapidity of performing the examination in a few minutes.
> No appreciable delay between a decision to obtain the examination and the results of the test.
> Simplicity and economy in performing the examination.
> Acceptance by physicians and patients.
> Ability to perform examination in an operated or traumatised extremity.
> Ability to obtain information about the competency of deep venous valves.

The disadvantages of the procedure are:
> High false negative findings if the calf veins alone are involved.
> Inability to detect thrombi in the pelvic veins.

On balance, the procedure is very suitable for mass application in screening and surveillance provided its limitations are borne in mind.

REFERENCES

Sigel, B. et al. (1968) *Surg., Gynec. and Obstet.*, **127,** 339.
Sigel, B. et al. (1970) *Arch. Surg.*, **100,** 535.
Thorner, R. M. and Remein, Q. R. (1961) *P.H.S. Publ. No.* 846. Washington D.C.: U.S. Government Printing Office.

9 Isotopic Detection of Deep Venous Thrombosis

V. V. Kakkar

There can be little doubt of the importance of deep vein thrombosis of the lower limbs and its consequences. Pulmonary embolus is now one of the commonest causes of death following surgery; not only is it relatively frequent in prostrating medical illness (Bailey and Beavan, 1969), but it is the greatest single factor in maternal mortality in childbirth (Beller, 1968). Apart from the immediate risk to life, there are the late sequelae following destruction of venous valves, of swelling of the legs, varicose veins, ulceration and other trophic changes. These represent one of the commonest and most intractable problems in surgery.

The difficulty in assessing the frequency of deep vein thrombosis has been the absence of any practical means for recognising the condition accurately. If one relies solely on clinical signs, the condition will remain undiagnosed in about half of the patients (Flanc et al., 1968). If fatal pulmonary embolus is regarded as the only definite evidence of preceding venous thrombosis, then in 95 per cent of such cases the disease may be clinically 'silent' (Welch and Faxen, 1941). During the last few years a number of tests have been developed which can be used for the detection of deep vein thrombosis. These include the ^{125}I-labelled fibrinogen test, the ultrasound technique and the electrical impedance method. The introduction of modern diagnostic X-ray equipment, including the image intensifier and television monitor screen, has also permitted us to demonstrate with greater precision than ever before the deep veins of the legs and the presence or absence of thrombosis there. This has made it possible to confirm the accuracy of the new methods of detecting thrombi.

The role of the electrical impedance test, the ultrasound technique and phlebography in diagnosing venous thrombi is discussed by other authors. A brief description of the ^{125}I-labelled fibrinogen test and its usefulness as a diagnostic tool is presented in this paper.

DEVELOPMENT OF ^{125}I-LABELLED FIBRINOGEN TEST

Hobbs and Davies (1960) first showed experimentally that there is preferential uptake of ^{131}I-labelled fibrinogen by a forming thrombus, and suggested that this might serve as the basis of a valuable clinical test for the detection of early thrombi. Later, Palko et al. (1964) used the test to confirm the presence of deep vein thrombosis suspected on clinical grounds. Unfortunately, there were many defects in the use of this isotope. Atkins and Hawkins (1965) substituted the isotope ^{125}I for ^{131}I in labelling the fibrinogen because of its many advantages. The isotope ^{125}I emits a soft gamma radiation and therefore the apparatus used for detecting radioactivity can be lighter and more mobile. This has allowed us to develop light and portable equipment which can be used at the patient's bedside (Kakkar et al., 1970). Secondly, the longer half-life (60 days) of ^{125}I leads to a greater differential between thrombus and surrounding tissue, since catabolism of fibrinogen is unaffected by the isotope used; there is also the practical advantage of a longer shelf life. Thirdly, the total body radiation with ^{125}I is less than that with ^{131}I; although the thyroid gland receives a slightly higher dose, this is at a much slower rate. The only disadvantage is that tissue absorption with ^{125}I is greater than with ^{131}I; for example, at a depth of 3 cm, ^{131}I gives 50 per cent of the surface count, while ^{125}I emits only 23 per cent.

LABELLING OF FIBRINOGEN

Human fibrinogen, in the form of anti-haemophilic factor concentrate (Kabi), has been used. In order to minimise any possible risk of transmitting viral hepatitis, special precautions are taken in the preparation of the fibrinogen. It is obtained from a restricted pool of accredited donors.

Carrier-free ^{125}I in sodium hydroxide solution, with a specific activity of 20 millicuries per ml, is obtained from the Radiochemical Centre, Amersham, England. The fibrogen is iodinated using the 'jet iodination' method of McFarlane (1963). Free iodine is reduced to less than 5 per cent of the total iodine by passing the solution through a pyrogen-free resin column (Amberlite IRA–400). Ten millicuries of ^{125}I are usually used to iodinate 60 mg of fibrinogen. The efficiency of labelling usually varies between 30 to 60 per cent. The labelled fibrinogen and the solutions used in its preparation are stored at $-20°$C. The sterility of the labelled fibrinogen is checked frequently.

TEST PROCEDURE

The test can be used in every type of patient: surgical, orthopaedic, obstetric and medical. In surgical patients, the thyroid gland is blocked by sodium iodide (100 mg) given orally, in order to prevent excessive uptake of radioactive iodine. Twenty-four hours later, on the day before operation, 100 μci of ^{125}I-labelled fibrinogen are injected intravenously. In postpartum patients the sodium iodide can be given intravenously immediately after delivery and ^{125}I-labelled fibrinogen is injected half an hour later. Similarly, in medical patients—those with myocardial infarction, for example, the thyroid gland can be blocked as soon as the patient is confined

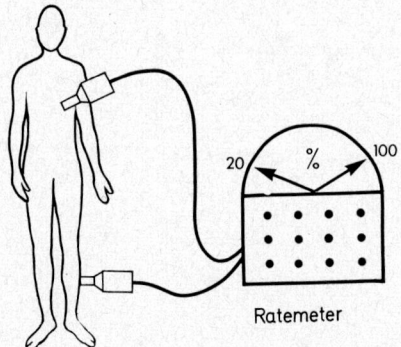

FIG. 9.1. The principle of the ratemeter; the readings on the linear scale are a direct percentage of the heart count.

to bed. ^{125}I-labelled fibrinogen (100 μci) is injected into an arm vein and the radioactivity over the legs is measured two hours later.

The older method of counting radioactivity, where absolute counts were obtained at each position in the limb (Flanc *et al.*, 1968), has now been superseded by a much simpler and faster technique, using a ratemeter (Kakkar *et al.*, 1970). The scintillation counter is first placed over the precordial region (a site marked in the fourth left intercostal space) and the radioactivity over the heart measured, the machine being adjusted to represent a reading of 100 per cent. All subsequent readings on the linear scale of the ratemeter are a direct percentage of the heart count (Fig. 9.1). For measuring radioactivity, the legs are elevated on an adjustable stand to decrease venous pooling and give access to the calf for the scintillation counter. Counting is performed along the thigh and calf positions which have been marked at two-inch intervals (Fig. 9.2). The readings are then recorded directly from the machine, without calculations, as shown in Table 9.1.

An increase of more than 20 in the percentage value was found on the 2nd post-operative day, in the right calf at positions 3 and 4, and this persisted for several days. At the same time, a similar rise

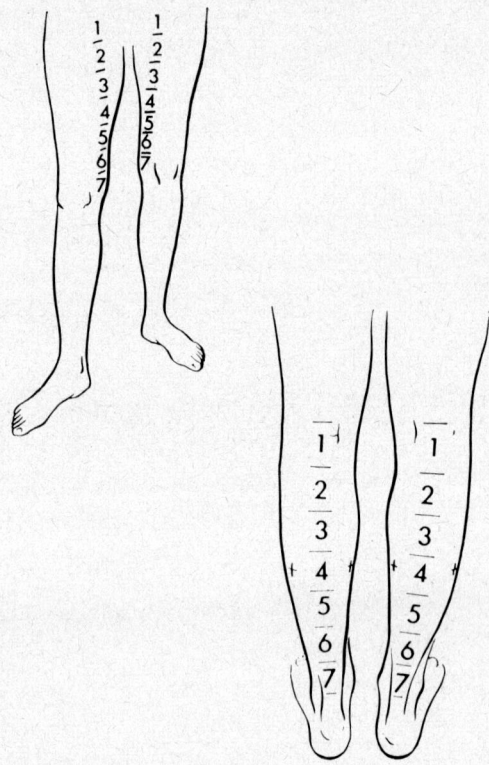

Fig. 9.2. Positions at which the radioactivity is measured.

in readings was found in the left calf at position 3 on the 1st post-operative day. On subsequent days, there were increases in readings at positions 4 and 5, indicating that the thrombus was spreading.

After counting one limb, the scintillation counter is placed over the same area in the precordial region to check any 'drift' in the machine. The time required to count both limbs is 10 to 12 minutes. Counting is carried out before operation and this is taken as a baseline for comparison with subsequent counts. Radioactivity is again measured thereafter at daily intervals. In practice, it is probably

TABLE 9.1
INDIVIDUAL RADIOACTIVITY READINGS IN A CASE OF VENOUS THROMBOSIS

Leg positions	Percentage of heart count						
	Pre-op.	Post-op.	Days after operation				
			1	2	3	4	5
Right leg: Thigh							
1	52	61	48	43	50	64	55
2	47	56	41	40	43	56	52
3	42	47	37	38	41	46	50
4	37	42	33	39	36	44	48
5	36	39	30	36	31	40	86
Calf							
1	37	49	38	40	34	40	90
2	33	50	30	44	42	60	110
3	33	46	33	57	64	70	120
4	30	40	35	58	60	80	88
5	29	34	31	40	36	40	72
6						30	
Left leg: Thigh							
1	39	54	34	35	40	34	27
2	38	49	32	32	36	33	28
3	36	42	27	20	34	32	30
4	33	42	24	29	31	33	37
5	30	34	24	28	33	32	36
Calf							
1	30	51	34	36	38	36	52
2	27	46	37	60	39	46	66
3	26	46	65	88	115	120	120
4	26	40	30	102	65	120	120
5	26	34	24	50	34	60	90
6				30	26	30	48

sufficient to carry out counts pre-operatively and on the first, third and sixth post-operative days; if there are indications of a forming thrombus, then counting can be performed daily, to see whether the thrombus is increasing or dissolving.

It has been shown that an increase in the percentage value of 20 or more represents the formation of a thrombus in the deep veins of the legs (Kakkar *et al.*, 1970).

The ratemeter (Fig. 9.3) has many advantages over the older method of counting radioactivity. It is just as accurate in detecting a thrombus and can be used to follow its course, whether it is extending, remaining unchanged or being lysed. The apparatus is portable

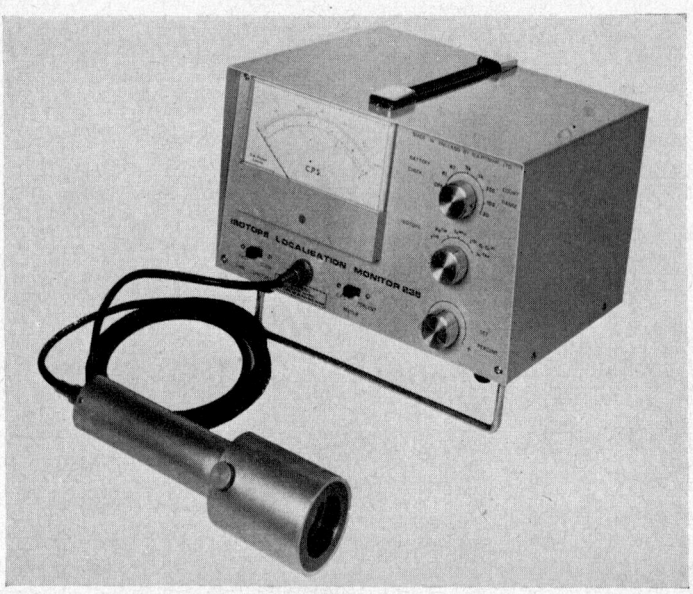

FIG. 9.3. Ratemeter (Pitman Model 235 isotope localisation monitor) and scintillation counter.
(Reproduced from Kakkar *et al.* (1970) by courtesy of the Editor of the *Lancet*).

and much simpler to use than the older method. A physiotherapist or technician alone can scan and record readings accurately.

ACCURACY OF ^{125}I-LABELLED FIBRINOGEN TEST AS A SCREENING PROCEDURE

The accuracy of the radioactive fibrinogen test in diagnosing deep vein thrombosis has been confirmed by ascending functional phlebography. In 88 patients, both the radioactive fibrinogen test and phlebographic examination were used in each case to confirm the presence or absence of deep vein thrombosis. The findings of both tests agreed in 82 patients, that is, in approximately 92 per cent (Table 9.2).

Table 9.2

CORRELATION OF PHLEBOGRAPHIC FINDINGS WITH ^{125}I-FIBRINOGEN TEST IN 88 PATIENTS

^{125}I-fibrinogen test	Phlebography	Total
+ve	+ve	32 ⎫ 82
−ve	−ve	50 ⎭
+ve	−ve	4
−ve	+ve	2
		88

Both tests agreed in 82/88 = 92%.

Both tests were positive in 32 patients, negative in 50, and in 4 patients the radioactive fibrinogen test was positive while phlebograms failed to show thrombi. The failure of X-rays to show thrombi in these 4 patients may be due to the fact that the thrombi were confined to the muscular veins of the calf, which are difficult to demonstrate by phlebographic examination. In 2 patients, the radioactive fibrinogen test was negative but the phlebograms showed a filling defect in the tibial veins, which probably represented old thrombi.

RESULTS OF CLINICAL STUDIES

The ^{125}I-labelled fibrinogen test has now been recognised as a suitable method for the routine screening of 'at risk' patients, and also for confirmation of the diagnosis in those patients who present with clinical features suggestive of deep vein thrombosis.

Use of ^{125}I-fibrinogen test as routine screening procedure. We have used this test in 799 patients in order to detect venous thrombi at their earliest stages and to determine the true incidence of this condition in various groups of patients. The results of some of these studies are presented here. The studies in surgical patients are presented in detail. Those from initial studies of other groups of patients are referred to, and are presented in detail by Field *et al.* (page 117).

Surgical patients. In 469 consecutive patients aged 40 or over, admitted to hospital for elective surgery, the ^{125}I-labelled fibrinogen test was used as a routine screening procedure. Patients who had a history or clinical signs of recent deep vein thrombosis and those undergoing leg or thyroid operations were excluded. Of these patients, 130 (27·8 per cent) developed deep vein thrombosis; in older patients undergoing major operations, there was an even greater incidence of over 50 per cent. In 68 patients (52·3 per cent), thrombi formed during operation or within the first 24 hours, while in the remaining 62 (47·7 per cent) the increased radioactive counts developed within three to seven days after operation. In the majority of patients (66·1 per cent) the process affected only one limb (Table 9.3).

In a prospective study of 203 surgical patients (Kakkar et al., 1970), the radioactive fibrinogen test was used to assess the value of clinical signs in the diagnosis of venous thrombosis. Patients were examined every day and particular attention was paid to any tenderness in the calf, the presence or absence of ankle oedema and a rise in skin temperature; the circumference of the lower limbs was

TABLE 9.3

INCIDENCE OF DEEP VEIN THROMBOSIS IN 469 SURGICAL PATIENTS

	Number of patients
Deep vein thrombosis	130 (27·8%)
Bilateral	44 (33·9%)
Unilateral	86 (66·1%)
Right leg	42
Left leg	34

measured at various levels. If clinical signs suggestive of pulmonary embolism developed, a chest X-ray and electrocardiogram were performed and repeated on subsequent days. In some patients, lung scanning was also performed, using macroaggregated ferric chloride labelled with indium^{113m}.

Despite this careful examination, only 30 of the 62 patients in whom deep vein thrombosis developed showed any clinical signs. Local tenderness and/or mild ankle oedema was present in only 37 of the 86 limbs with raised counts. Tenderness in the calf was detected in 27 of the 86 legs and corresponded roughly with the area of increased radioactivity. Mild ankle oedema alone was present in the other 10 limbs. Whenever clinical signs did appear, the radioactive test anticipated the onset of thrombosis by at least 24 to 36 hours. In 6 of the 62 patients with proven thrombosis, symptoms and signs of pulmonary embolism developed and in only 2 of these could clinical signs of deep vein thrombosis be demonstrated in the legs.

The calf was by far the most common site of increased radioactivity (89·5 per cent) and only infrequently (10·5 per cent) did increased radioactivity commence in the popliteal fossa or over the lower half of the thigh (Table 9.4).

In those patients where the raised counts were observed over the calf region, phlebograms showed normal femoral and iliac veins.

Orthopaedic patients. Of 50 patients investigated, 27 (54 per cent) developed deep vein thrombosis. It was interesting to note that in 17 limbs (34 per cent) which had not sustained trauma, thrombosis also developed. Twenty-eight per cent of patients had bilateral deep vein thrombosis. A much higher incidence was observed in those patients who had pertrochanteric fractures when compared with those who had sub-capital fractures.

This difference could be due to the greater severity of injury and the longer time required for operation in patients with pertrochanteric fractures.

TABLE 9.4

POST-OPERATIVE DEEP VEIN THROMBOSIS—SITE OF RAISED COUNTS

Site	No. of legs
Calf	77 (89·5%)
Popliteal fossa	5
Lower half of thigh	4
Upper half of thigh	0
Total	86

Urological patients. Ten of 42 patients studied developed deep vein thrombosis, giving an overall incidence of 23·8 per cent. The incidence of thrombosis was much lower in the 24 patients subjected to transurethral resection.

Trauma from transurethral resection is less than that following 'open' operation, and stasis in the calf veins is reduced during transurethral resection because the legs are elevated. These two factors may explain the low incidence of venous thrombosis in this group.

Obstetric patients. In a group of 80 patients who had normal deliveries, 3 developed deep vein thrombosis. None was found in a group of 20 patients who underwent Caesarian section (Friend and Kakkar, 1970).

Gynaecological patients. The overall incidence of deep vein thrombosis in 92 gynaecological patients over the age of 30 years was 18·4 per cent. This low incidence, as compared with that seen in general surgical patients, may be due to their being relatively young females who were not generally ill at the time of operation. Only one of the 17 cases of deep vein thrombosis occurred in a patient who had undergone vaginal surgery in the lithotomy position, although 36 per cent of the patients were in this position during operation.

Myocardial infarction patients. In a study of 52 patients admitted to the coronary intensive care unit, a diagnosis of myocardial infarction was confirmed in 31 patients. Eighteen of these were treated with anticoagulants. Six of the 31 patients (19 per cent) developed deep vein thrombosis, 5 of these belonging to the group of 13 who did not receive anticoagulants.

It was observed that there was a high incidence (62 per cent) of venous thrombosis in patients who were 'severely ill', whatever the cause. Similar findings have been reported by other workers (Murray *et al.*, 1970).

^{125}I-FIBRINOGEN TEST AND 'ESTABLISHED' THROMBOSIS

The usefulness of the ^{125}I-labelled fibrinogen test in confirming diagnosis in those patients who present with suggestive symptoms and signs has also been investigated. Deep vein thrombosis was suspected in 82 patients on the basis of clinical examination; they were arbitrarily classified in three clinical groups: those with minimal signs, those with major signs and those with signs of a massive thrombosis (Table 9.5).

TABLE 9.5

^{125}I-FIBRINOGEN TEST AND PHLEBOGRAPHY IN LEGS WITH CLINICAL SIGNS OF THROMBOSIS

	No. of legs	^{125}I-fibrinogen test positive	Phlebogram positive
Minor signs	35	26	24
Major signs	42	34	29
Massive signs	25	16	21
Total	102	76	74

The radioactive fibrinogen test and ascending functional phlebography (Kakkar and Flanc, 1968) were used for diagnostic assessment in each case. The procedure of the radioactive fibrinogen test was similar to that already described. A positive diagnosis of deep vein thrombosis was made if the counts became raised over the limb and persisted; the exact criteria for diagnosing the presence of thrombosis are discussed in detail elsewhere (Flanc et al., 1968).

Group I: Minimal signs. Twenty-four patients had local tenderness in the calf, or mild oedema at the ankle, or both tenderness and oedema. Phlebography was performed in 35 limbs and thrombi were seen in 24. Eleven had normal veins. The radioactive counts were raised in 26 limbs but were normal in 9. In 4 patients, both the ^{125}I-labelled fibrinogen test and phlebography were negative. These patients were assumed not to have thrombosis.

Group II: Major signs. There were 33 patients in this group. Deep vein thrombosis was suspected in each because they all showed marked tenderness of the calf muscles or in the popliteal fossa; they had ankle oedema or there was an obvious increase in the temperature of the leg. Phlebography was performed in 42 limbs and was positive in 29, negative in 12 and the examination failed in one limb. The radioactive fibrinogen test was positive in 34 limbs and negative in 8. In 6 patients phlebograms did not show thrombi. Of these, one patient had cellulitis of the leg, one had ruptured the medial head of gastrocnemius and one, who had sustained a fractured ankle, developed oedema and tenderness when the plaster cast was removed. In the other 3 patients, the cause of the physical signs was unexplained.

Group III: Massive signs. There were 23 patients in this group. They presented with acute swelling of the whole limb and tenderness over the entire course of the femoral vein in the thigh. Eight patients had, in addition, cyanotic discoloration of the foot. Phlebography was performed in 25 limbs and was positive in 21. In 2 patients, who were in congestive cardiac failure, exacerbation of the symptoms was due to acute atrial occlusion and in both the phlebograms were normal.

DISCUSSION

The diagnosis of deep vein thrombosis presents two separate problems. One is that of diagnosing occult or asymptomatic thrombi; for this, a quick, simple and accurate screening procedure is required, which can be used in a large number of patients who are at risk of developing this condition. The second problem is entirely different: how best to confirm diagnosis in patients who present with clinical features suggestive of deep vein thrombosis. Of all the methods which are now available, including the ultrasound test (Strandness et al., 1967; Sigel et al., 1968), the electrical impedance technique (Mullick et al., 1970) and phlebography, the radioactive fibrinogen test would seem to be ideal for use as a routine screening procedure to investigate all types of patients (medical, obstetric and surgical), as clearly demostrated by the findings reported in this paper and by a number of other studies (Negus et al., 1968; Atkins and Hawkins, 1968; Lambie et al., 1970; Murray et al., 1970; Pinto, 1970 and others).

The advantages of using the radioactive fibrinogen test as a screening procedure are that it is quick, safe and accurate. The accuracy of this method in detecting thrombi in the legs was shown by ascending functional phlebography (Kakkar and Flanc, 1968) and later confirmed by several workers (Negus et al., 1968; Lambie et al., 1970, and others). Using this test, we have found that there is a great advantage in detecting thrombosis in all patients at the earliest possible stage (Kakkar et al., 1969b, c) and that the progress of the thrombus must be followed to see if it is extending, remaining unchanged or lysing. The various forms of treatment at present available are neither simple nor safe, and their administration cannot be justified in every patient who develops thrombosis (Kakkar et al., 1969b). It has been shown that only when the thrombotic process extends from the calf into the more proximal veins, including the popliteal, femoral and pelvic veins, is there a high risk of pulmonary embolism (Kakkar et al., 1969c). This extension of the thrombus can be easily detected by the method described, and treatment can be instituted at the proper time.

There are three theoretical disadvantages of using the radioactive fibrinogen technique. One is the problem of detecting a thrombus in the upper third of the thigh and pelvis. Diagnosis by this method depends on a sufficient difference between the radioactivity in the thrombus and in its surrounding background. In the upper thigh and pelvis, the proximity of the bladder, containing radioactive urine, and large arteries and other vascular structures gives an increased background count which makes the test less reliable in these situations.

The failure of the test to detect iliac vein thrombosis is clearly a disadvantage but it is of little clinical significance because thrombi rarely start in this region, and it is unusual for thrombosis to occur in the thigh or pelvis without concurrent thrombosis of the calf veins. These findings, though different from those reported by Sevitt et al. (1962), are supported by a number of other autopsy reports (Neumann 1938; Frykholm, 1939) and phlebographic studies (Bauer, 1940, 1964), and recent studies where the radioactive fibrinogen test and ascending functional phlebography have been used to detect the development of venous thrombi and to follow their course accurately.

The second disadvantage is that this test carries a risk of serum hepatitis because of the administration of fibrinogen. This risk, however, can be minimised or eliminated by taking special precautions in the preparation of the fibrinogen. This should be obtained from a small pool of donors who have donated blood for at least five previous transfusions without clinical evidence of viral hepatitis occurring in the recipients in the succeeding six months, each batch being screened for Australian Antigen. In our present studies, this type of fibrinogen has been used in over 800 patients and not a single case of clinical serum hepatitis has occurred.

The only real disadvantage of the test concerns the manpower required to carry it out. Since in every hospital there are large numbers of patients at risk of developing deep vein thrombosis, it would seem impossible to screen each and every one by this method. This would be a valid argument if the original method of measuring radioactivity (Atkins and Hawkins, 1965; Flanc et al., 1968; Negus et al., 1968), where the counting and calculating of results took a considerable time, was still being used. The apparatus was heavy, cumbersome and expensive and skilled staff were needed to obtain accurate results. However, most of these disadvantages have been overcome with the introduction of the ratemeter (Kakkar et al., 1970). The scanning time has been reduced from about half an hour to less than 15 minutes and the readings are obtained directly from a linear scale on the ratemeter, thus eliminating the need for lengthy calculations. The ratemeter is portable and simple to use—a physiotherapist or a technician alone can scan and record readings accurately. If it is not possible to screen each and every patient, this should at least be used in those patients who are at a greater risk of developing deep vein thrombosis, in other words, the 'high risk' group.

Despite these drawbacks, the radioactive fibrinogen test remains a quick, safe and accurate method for detecting early and forming thrombi. It is ideal for use as a routine screening procedure for the investigation of large numbers of patients.

What is the value of the radioactive fibrinogen test as a diagnostic tool for use in patients who present with some clinical signs of thrombosis? A positive result will be obtained only if a thrombus is still forming; once thrombi are fully established, the test may be negative. Although a negative result was obtained in one-sixth of the limbs, the radioactive test was succcessful in diagnosing thrombosis in the majority of cases. In our studies, it proved to be a valuable diagnostic tool, particularly in those patients with minor clinical signs, because it was in this group that clinical diagnosis was most fallible. There is a further advantage of using this test in such patients: whenever the test is positive, it provides a simple method of assessing the effectiveness of treatment (Kakkar et al., 1969a and b). By observing the change in radioactivity at the site of a thrombus, it is possible to tell whether the thrombus is extending, remaining unchanged or being lysed.

The ^{125}I-labelled fibrinogen test has also proved to be of great value in research, since it is the only objective method for detecting early and forming thrombi, thus enabling accurate assessment to be made in studies of treatment (Kakkar et al., 1969a, b), and prophylaxis (Flanc et al., 1969; Kakkar et al., 1970; Pinto, 1970; Browse and Negus, 1970; Lambie et al., 1970; Rosengarten et al., 1970) of this condition.

The problems of deep vein thrombosis and its management can be fairly likened to an iceberg: only the tip—the overt manifestations of gross thrombosis—have been recognised in the past. Now, sensitive and precise techniques have been developed for the recognition and measurement of a thrombus. In most cases, thrombosis starts in the calf veins and when it extends proximally, active treatment is required. In this situation, there is a significant risk of pulmonary embolism (Kakkar et al., 1969a) and when long segments of veins are involved, there is considerable danger of the development of the post-phlebitic syndrome. Thus it is clearly important in all patients to detect thrombosis at an early stage and to follow its course. This requires a simple method which can be used in most hospitals. Neither the ultrasound technique nor the impedance test can detect early thrombi which start in the muscular veins of the calf or in the tibial veins, nor can they be used to follow the course of thrombi accurately. The ^{125}I-labelled fibrinogen test, however, goes a long way towards fulfilling these requirements.

ACKNOWLEDGEMENT

Material and figures presented in this paper have been reproduced from the article: 'Use of Radioactive Fibrogen in Diagnosis of venous Thrombosis'. From *Archives of Surgery*, February 1972, by kind permission of the editor.

REFERENCES

ATKINS, P. and HAWKINS, L. A. (1965) *Lancet*, **2**, 1217.
BAILEY, R. R. and BEAVAN, D. W. (1969).
BAUER, G. (1940) *Acta Chir. Scand.*, **84**, Suppl. 61.
BAUER, G. (1964) *Am. J. Cardiol.*, **14**, 29.
BELLER, F. K. (1968) *Brit. J. Surg.*, **55**, 742.
BROWSE, N. and NEGUS, D. (1970) *Brit. med. J.*, **3**, 615.
FLANC, C. et al. (1968) *Brit. J. Surg.*, **55**, 742.
FLANC, C. et al. (1969) *Lancet*, **1**, 477.

FRIEND, J. R. and KAKKAR, V. V. (1970) *J. Obst. Gynaec. Brit. Cwlth*, **77,** 820.
FRYKHOLM, R. (1939) *Nord. Med.*, **4,** 3534.
HOBB, J. T. and DAVIES, J. W. L. (1960) *Lancet*, **2,** 134.
KAKKAR, V. V. and FLANC, C. (1968) *Brit. J. Surg.*, **55,** 384.
KAKKAR, V. V. (1969) *Ann. Roy. Coll. Surg. Engl.*, **45,** 257.
KAKKAR, V. V. et al. (1969a) *Lancet*, **2,** 230.
KAKKAR, V. V. et al. (1969b) *Brit. med. J.* **1,** 806.
KAKKAR, V. V. et al. (1969c) *Brit. J. Surg.*, **56,** 178.
KAKKAR, V. V. (1970) *Proc. Roy. Soc. Med.*, **63,** 133.
KAKKAR, V. V. et al. (1970) *Lancet*, **1,** 540.
LAMBIE, J. M. et al. (1970) *Brit. med. J.*, **2,** 142.
MCFARLANE, A. S. (1963) *J. Clin. Invest.* **42,** 346.
MULLICK, S. C. et al. (1970) *Am. J. Surg.* **119,** 417.
MURRAY, T. S. et al. (1970) *Lancet*, **2,** 792.
NEGUS, D. et al. (1968) *Brit. J. Surg.*, **55,** 835.
NEUMANN, R. (1938) *Virch. Arch.*, **301,** 708.
PALKO, P. D. et al. (1964) *Can. J. Surg.*, **7,** 215.
PINTO, D. J. (1970) *Brit. J. Surg.*, **57,** 349.
ROSENGARTEN, D. S. et al. (1970) *Brit. J. Surg.*, **57,** 296.
SEVITT, S. et al. (1962) *Am. J. Med.*, **33,** 703.
SIGEL, B. et al. (1968) *Surg. Gynec. Obstet.*, **127,** 339.
STRANDNESS, D. E. et al. (1967) *Am. J. Surg.*, **113,** 311.
WELCH, C. E. and FAXEN, H. H. (1941).

10 Deep Vein Thrombosis after Myocardial Infarction, Prostatectomy and Fracture of the Femoral Neck

E. S. Field, V. V. Kakkar and A. N. Nicolaides

INTRODUCTION

The results of three studies, in each of which the ^{125}I-labelled fibrinogen test was employed to investigate the incidence of deep vein thrombosis, are reported here. In each study, the patients present a separate problem.

The theory and technique of the ^{125}I-fibrinogen test which has revolutionised research into the subject of deep vein thrombosis has been described (Kakkar and Howe, page 101). It is a method that is at once objective and precise yet, since the development of the ratemeter, simple. It has confirmed that clinical signs are a wholly unreliable guide to the presence and extent of deep vein thrombosis (Flanc et al., 1968), so that much otherwise excellent work hitherto published on the subject has been invalidated. It has become necessary to reinvestigate many of the baffling problems in order to establish true statistics concerning the incidence of deep vein thrombosis. Apart from incidence, the test can be used as a tool in determining the aetiological factors responsible for deep venous thrombosis, can detect the site of origin and natural history of the thrombotic process and, finally, can be used for testing the efficacy of proposed measures of prophylaxis and even treatment of the established disease.

In the trial carried out in the Coronary Care Unit at King's College Hospital (Nicolaides et al., 1971) it was proposed to investigate the incidence of deep vein thrombosis in a group of patients known from previous clinical and autopsy studies (Hilden et al., 1961; Browder et al., 1959; M.R.C. Report, 1969) to be a 'high-risk' group with regard to both fatal and non-fatal thromboembolic phenomena. It became possible in this small pilot study to demonstrate the beneficial effect of anticoagulants (as a result of which a further prospective, randomised trial is now underway), and to establish a sub-group of patients with a particularly high incidence of deep vein thrombosis.

The study of patients undergoing prostatectomy was again prompted by previous reports of a high incidence following this operation (Antila *et al.*, 1965; Becker *et al.*, 1970). It was hoped that factors such as operative trauma and posture during the operation might also be investigated.

The third study reported here was carried out on fifty patients admitted with fractures of the neck of the femur. Once again a known 'high-risk' group was chosen for investigation. It was necessary here to show first that the test was valid in these patients with lower limb injuries and the resultant extravasation of blood and radioactive fibrin. Obviously such extravascular radioactivity interferes with accurate scanning by the counter above the knee. However, we were able to demonstrate by using venography in all patients that thrombi were always detectable originally in the calf, where the test is accurate. Having done this it was possible to demonstrate the high incidence of deep venous thrombosis in the group as a whole, but particularly in patients with a pertrochanteric fracture.

CORONARY CARE UNIT TRIAL

In the 1969 Medical Research Council Report, post-mortem studies revealed an incidence of 8·3 per cent pulmonary emboli in patients dying after myocardial infarction. Similar results had previously been obtained by the Medical Research Council, as well as in a series at King's College Hospital of 240 patients dying after myocardial infarction where an incidence of 7·9 per cent pulmonary emboli causing, or contributing to, death was recorded (Nicolaides, 1970). This trial was prompted by these findings.

MATERIALS AND METHODS

Fifty-two patients admitted with severe chest pain to the Coronary Care Unit were studied. All had been well prior to admission. Any patient under 40 years or with a history of recent venous thrombosis or pulmonary embolism was excluded from the trial. In 31 of the 52 patients the diagnosis of myocardial infarction was confirmed by E.C.G. and enzyme studies. The other 21 proved to have other causes of chest pain: pneumonia, hiatus hernia with oesophagitis and even one case of dissecting aneurysm. No patient was thought or found to have pulmonary embolus.

Of the 31 patients with myocardial infarction, 18 were treated with anticoagulants (intravenous heparin infusion 10,000 i.u. every 6 hours for 36 hours and immediate commencement of oral anticoagulants aimed at keeping the prothrombin time $1\frac{1}{2}$–2 times normal). Otherwise all myocardial infarction patients were treated identically. The use of anticoagulants was not randomised but was decided by the usual practice of the physician under whose care the patient had been admitted.

Each patient was given 100 mg sodium iodide daily for 30 days, and within 24 hours of admission received 100 μci radioactive fibrinogen. Radioactive counting with the Pitman 235 monitor was commenced after labelling, and thereafter carried out on alternate days or daily if thrombosis was suggested by the counts—the criteria for a diagnosis of thrombosis, together with further methodological details, have been described by Kakkar, page 101.

Results: Tables 10.1–10.3.

TABLE 10.1

PATIENTS INVESTIGATED—SHOWING OVERALL INCIDENCE IN TWO GROUPS

	Myocardial infarction	*Other causes Chest pain*	*Total*
No. of patients	31	21	52
No. with D.V.T.	6	2	8
% with D.V.T.	19%	9·9%	

TABLE 10.2

PATIENTS WITH MYOCARDIAL INFARCTION SHOWING EFFECT OF ANTICOAGULANTS ON INCIDENCE

	No anticoagulants	*Anticoagulants*	*Total*
No. of patients	13	18	31
No. with D.V.T.	5	1	6
% with D.V.T.	38%	5·5%	19%

TABLE 10.3

All patients subdivided into 'severely ill' and normotensive groups, showing that 62% of the severely ill group develop D.V.T. but only 7% of the other group. These 7% are bed-bound, non-anticoagulated patients with infarcts.

SEVERELY ILL GROUP

	No anticoagulants	Anticoagulants	Chest pain ? cause	Total
No. of patients	2	2	4	8
No. with D.V.T.	2	1	2	5 (62%)

NORMOTENSIVE GROUP

	No anticoagulants	Anticoagulants	Chest pain ? cause	Total
No. of patients	11	16	17	44
No. with D.V.T.	3	0	0	3 (7%)

Six of 31 patients with myocardial infarction (19 per cent) developed deep vein thrombosis. Only 2 of the other group of miscellaneous causes of chest pain developed deep venous thrombosis. Of the 6 patients with deep vein thrombosis in the myocardial infarction group, 5 were not anticoagulated and the other, though receiving anticoagulants, was classed as 'severely ill'. This meant that they were hypotensive with low cardiac output, poor peripheral circulation and reduced urinary production for 24 hours or more. The incidence in this group was 62 per cent while in the normotensive group regardless of diagnosis or anticoagulants it was 7 per cent.

Judged by the radioisotope counts none of the thrombi extended into the popliteal or other proximal veins and there were no overt pulmonary emboli.

DISCUSSION

Two facts emerge from the reported figures. One is the low incidence of deep vein thrombosis when anticoagulants are used for myocardial infarction. The other is the low incidence in patients whose blood pressure returns rapidly to normal. Indeed in the 16 normotensive patients treated with anticoagulants there was no case of deep vein thrombosis. All the thrombi occurred in patients who were hypotensive for prolonged periods or confined to bed without anticoagulants for the period of the investigation.

It must be conceded, however, that the figures in this pilot study are small and that a further prospective randomised trial on a larger number of patients is necessary. However, it should also be stressed that this study covers only the first 8–10 days after admission and therefore underestimates rather than exaggerates the incidence in patients kept at prolonged bed rest. The figures in this trial confirm those of other workers (Murray et al., 1970).

The importance of establishing this incidence lies not in the figures themselves but in the fate of the thrombi detected. The radioactive counts show that thrombosis commences in the deep veins of the calf musculature. From this site a proportion will propagate into the proximal veins and a proportion of these will break off and be carried into the bloodstream as pulmonary emboli, some of which are fatal. In patients who are treated by bed rest stasis occurs, thus predisposing to deep vein thrombosis. It is important to detect this thrombosis early in order to treat it (a) by heparin and/or oral anticoagulants, to prevent propagation into proximal veins or, (b) by thrombolytic agents to promote clot dissolution. Much better, however, would be the prevention of deep venous thrombosis by the use of prophylactic anticoagulants. This trial, though limited, does show the benefit to be achieved by using anticoagulants routinely in patients confined to bed by myocardial infarction.

PROSTATECTOMY TRIAL

As had been mentioned earlier this study was prompted by recent reports based on venographic and autopsy findings (Antila et al., 1965; Becker et al., 1970) that deep vein thrombosis is common after prostatectomy and pulmonary embolism is the commonest cause of post-prostatectomy death. While post-mortem studies at this hospital do not confirm the latter view, it seemed necessary to investigate the former claim.

MATERIALS AND METHODS

Fifty consecutive patients undergoing routine prostatectomy were studied. They were aged between 55 and 92 years. Patients with a pre-operative history or evidence of recent venous thromboembolism were excluded.

Transurethral resection was performed in patients with obstructive urinary symptoms in whom the prostate gland was small and fibrous or benign and estimated to weigh less than 30 grams. It was used also for malignant prostates. Retropubic prostatectomy was reserved for larger glands thought clinically to be benign.

As in the previous study the diagnosis of deep vein thrombosis was made purely by the radioactive fibrinogen test, the accuracy of the test having been established elsewhere. Patients were labelled prior to operation and the legs scanned on alternate days or more regularly if thrombosis was suspected.

Results: Table 10.4.

TABLE 10.4

	Retropubic prostatectomy	Transurethral prostatectomy	Total
No. of patients	21	29	50
No. with D.V.T.	10	2	12
% with D.V.T.	47·6%	6·8%	24%

Of 50 patients studied, 12 (24 per cent) developed deep vein thrombosis. When analysed, however, these figures show that, of 21 patients undergoing retropubic prostatectomy, 10 (47·6 per cent) developed deep venous thrombosis, but only 2 of 29 (6·8 per cent) of those having transurethral resection developed this condition. The difference between these two groups is significant ($p = 0·001$). A study of the two groups with regard to the factors predisposing to deep venous thrombosis is of some interest. Both groups are similar in age, obesity and previous history of venous thromboembolism. However, 7 of the 29 patients undergoing transurethral resection had carcinoma proven histologically, whereas all prostates removed by retropubic operation were benign. None of these 7 patients developed deep vein thrombosis although previous studies have shown malignancy to be a predisposing factor.

In one of the 12 patients, the thrombus propagated into the popliteal vein, but in no patient was there overt evidence of pulmonary embolus.

DISCUSSION

Once again the figures in this pilot study are small but they do show a marked difference between patients undergoing retropubic prostatectomy and those having transurethral resection. Previous studies have shown deep venous thrombosis to be directly related to the severity of operative trauma (Kakkar *et al.*, 1970). Undoubtedly in this series, transurethral resection was a more minor operation;

the duration of operation, the quantity of prostatic tissue removed and the blood loss were all less than in retropubic prostatectomy.

Furthermore, the elevation of the legs into the lithotomy position for transurethral resection probably encouraged venous return by emptying the soleal veins by gravity. Additionally, the absence of post-operative pain after transurethral resection allowed earlier mobilisation of the patient with a relative reduction in venous stasis.

It must be stressed that early diagnosis is necessary if prevention of propagation is to be achieved, for it is the patient in whom thrombi propagate who is at risk of pulmonary embolism. The results suggest that if prophylactic measures are to be employed they should be directed at patients undergoing retropubic prostatectomy where the incidence is high (47·6 per cent).

ORTHOPAEDIC TRIAL

The patient with a fractured femoral neck runs a high risk of developing venous thromboembolism. This has been demonstrated by clinical (Sevitt and Gallagher, 1959), autopsy (Sevitt and Gallagher, 1959; Solonen, 1963) and venographic studies (Salzman et al., 1966; Stevens et al., 1968; Culver et al., 1970). Although the ^{125}I-fibrinogen test has been shown to be accurate and easy to use in surgical (Kakkar and Flanc, 1968; Negus et al., 1968), medical (Murray et al., 1970; Nicolaides et al., 1971), orthopaedic (Pinto, 1970), gynaecological (Friend and Kakkar, 1970) and postpartum (Friend, 1971) groups, the test is, however, unreliable in the region of the pelvis and over a wound or haematoma (Kakkar, 1969). These are important considerations in fractures of the femoral neck.

This study was designed with these facts in view, the main aim being to determine whether the radioactive fibrinogen test is of value in diagnosing deep vein thrombosis under these circumstances.

MATERIALS AND METHODS

Fifty patients who had sustained a subcapital or pertrochanteric fracture of the femur were studied. Forty-six were female, 4 male and their ages varied from 60 to 94 years (mean 74·2 years). All underwent internal fixation.

Within 24 hours of admission, each patient was started on sodium iodide 100 mg daily and received 100 μci of ^{125}I-labelled fibrinogen, after which external scintillation counting was commenced, as in previous trials. In all patients in this study a venogram was performed, using techniques described elsewhere. In 40 patients it was performed 6–9 days after admission, and in the remaining 10 patients it was carried out at 3–5 days. In 13 patients bilateral venography was performed. During the period of study no patient had overt evidence of pulmonary embolism. Three patients died from causes other than thromboembolic phenomena; they are not included in this series as full investigation by the radioactive test and venography had not been completed.

Results: Tables 10.5–10.8.

TABLE 10.5

INCIDENCE OF D.V.T. IN FRACTURED LIMBS AND IN THE OPPOSITE UNFRACTURED LIMBS

	Fractured limb	Unfractured limb
No. of patients	50	50
No. with D.V.T.	27	17
% with D.V.T.	54	34

TABLE 10.6

DIFFERENTIAL INCIDENCE OF D.V.T. IN FRACTURED LIMBS WHERE THE FRACTURE WAS: (A) PERTROCHANTERIC; (B) SUBCAPITAL

	Pertrochanteric fractures	Subcapital fractures
No. of patients	24	26
No. with D.V.T.	18	9
% with D.V.T.	75	34

TABLE 10.7

CORRELATION BETWEEN ^{125}I-FIBRINOGEN TEST AND VENOGRAPHY

^{125}I-fibrinogen test	Venography	No.
D.V.T.	D.V.T.	29
D.V.T.	Normal	7
Normal	Normal	25
Normal	D.V.T.	2

Table 10.5 shows the incidence of deep vein thrombosis in the fractured limbs (54 per cent) and in the unfractured limbs (34 per cent) detected by the ^{125}I-fibrinogen test. In 28 per cent the throm-

boses were bilateral. Table 10.6 shows furthermore that, if the fractures are subdivided into pertrochanteric and subcapital types, there is a much higher incidence in the former (75 per cent) than in the latter (34 per cent).

A comparison was made between the incidence of deep venous thrombosis determined by the ^{125}I-fibrinogen test and by venography in 63 limbs. Table 10.7 shows disagreement in 9 limbs, but in only 2 of these was the fibrinogen test negative when the venogram conclusively showed deep vein thrombosis. Table 10.8 gives a detailed account of these 9 limbs and offers explanations for the disagreement.

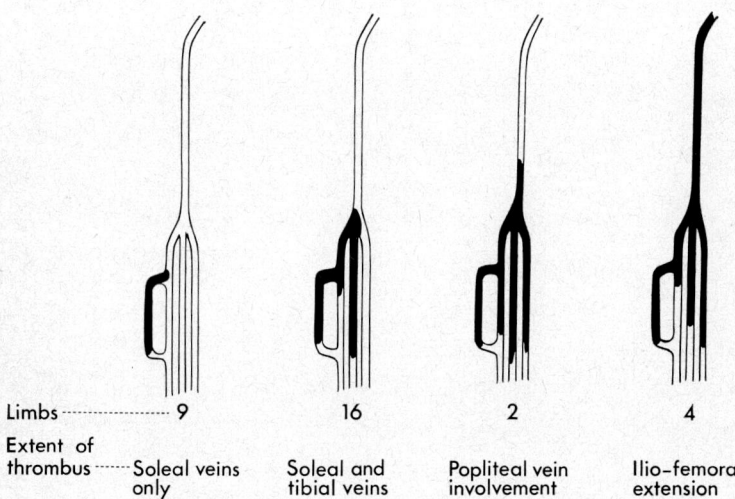

FIG. 10.1. Pattern and extent of thrombi in 31 venograms in which thrombosis was detected, showing number of limbs with each pattern. In the left diagram only the soleal veins are thrombosed. On the far right, soleal, tibial, popliteal and iliofemoral thrombosis has occurred.

Figure 10.1 shows the distribution and extent of the 31 thrombi found by venography, diagrammatically represented. In no case in this series was thrombosis *confined* to veins *above* the knee.

DISCUSSION

The results in this study indicate clearly that patients suffering from a fracture of the femoral neck form a 'high risk' group with respect to the development of deep vein thrombosis (54 per cent). Notable is the higher incidence in pertrochanteric (75 per cent) than in subcapital (34 per cent) fractures. Once again it is felt that this might be explained by the greater severity of operative trauma and of injury.

TABLE 10.8

REASONS FOR DISAGREEMENT BETWEEN FINDINGS OF VENOGRAPHY AND ^{125}I-FIBRINOGEN TEST IN 9 LIMBS

	^{125}I-fibrinogen test	Venography	Probable explanation
1.	Normal	Small tibial vein thrombus, with collaterals.	Old, non-extending thrombus
2.	Normal	Soleal vein thrombus	Non-extending thrombus
3.	Raised	N.A.D.	Superficial thrombophlebitis
4.	Raised	Poor venogram	Ankle oedema—inadequate X-rays
5.	Raised	N.A.D.	Superficial thrombophlebitis
6.	Raised	N.A.D.	Unable to elevate legs for scanning
7.	Raised	N.A.D.	Feeble patient—poor venogram
8.	Raised	N.A.D.	No obvious reason
9.	Raised	N.A.D.	No obvious reason

DISCUSSION

A major problem is the management of this group of patients with a high incidence of deep vein thrombosis, attendant risk to life from pulmonary embolism, and morbidity from the post-phlebitic sequelae. Dependence on clinical signs results in failure to diagnose the condition in about 50 per cent of patients (Kakkar and Flanc, 1968). A pulmonary embolus may be the first indication of venous thrombosis (Coon and Coller, 1959; Solonen, 1963; Freeark et al., 1967; Culver et al., 1970). Venography, although a most accurate method of detecting deep venous thrombosis, is not suitable as a screening method for large numbers of elderly patients. Ultrasonic techniques (Evans and Cockett, 1969), though relatively simple and causing the patient little disturbance, may not detect early, small, non-occlusive thrombi.

The ^{125}I-fibrinogen test has been shown to be accurate and able to detect thrombi at their earliest stage. Even in elderly people it can be used without much discomfort. In its latest form, employing the ratemeter, a technician can scan both limbs in less than 10 minutes. The major disadvantage of the radioactive fibrinogen test is its inaccuracy in the proximal femoral vein, the region of the pelvis or in the presence of an operation wound with extravasation of blood and radioactive fibrinogen; the external scintillation counter interprets extravascular and intravascular fibrin without discrimination.

Venography was performed in all our patients using techniques (Kakkar and Flanc, 1968; Nicolaides et al., 1971) which demonstrate calf veins and proximal veins as high as the inferior vena

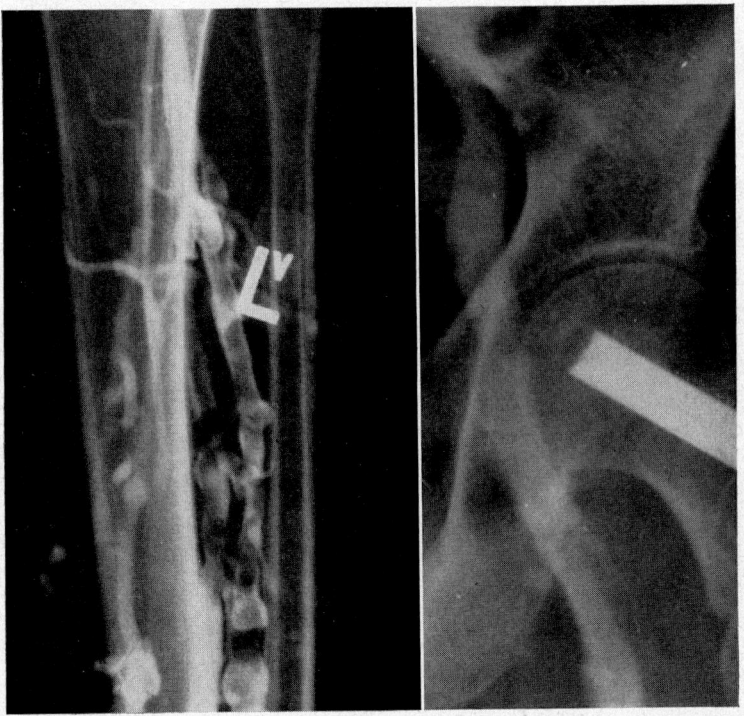

Fig. 10.2   Fig. 10.3

Fig. 10.2. Venogram showing extensive calf vein thrombosis.

Fig. 10.3. Venogram from same patient as Fig. 10.2, showing patient with normal iliofemoral segment. Trifin nail is seen.

cava (Figs. 10.2, 10.3). By combining the results of venography with those of the ^{125}I-fibrinogen test in 63 limbs we have shown that the site of origin of thrombi is in the calf despite the fact that the injury and operation are in the pelvic region. Venography at 3–5 days in a random small group of 10 patients convinced us that we were not missing transient thrombi, initiating the thrombotic process, in the large proximal veins. Thus the ^{125}I-fibrinogen test can be used where it is most accurate, in the calf, with the sure knowledge that it will detect the earliest thrombi.

These findings support those of many workers concerning the site of origin of thrombi (Frykholm, 1939; Bauer, 1940), but appear to be at variance with the views of others (Sevitt and Gallagher, 1959; Mavor and Galloway, 1969) who feel that, especially following hip trauma, a large number of thromboses arise within the large proximal veins. However, some of these studies are based on autopsy findings (Sevitt and Gallagher, 1959). This involves a highly selected group of patients, among which are many who have died some weeks after injury, with prolonged hypotension and widespread venous stasis.

The majority of patients with deep venous thrombosis survive, and it is in these patients that the dynamic process of venous thrombosis can be followed using the ^{125}I-fibrinogen test and repeated venography. From other, more extensive studies, the site of origin of thrombi in the calf has been established, as well as the significance of propagation of thrombi as source of pulmonary embolism. It has thus been one of the objects of this study to effect early diagnosis of deep vein thrombosis and to institute methods of preventing propagation (heparin and oral anticoagulants). However, trials of prophylactic measures currently in progress eventually should obviate the need for early detection.

CONCLUSIONS

Until 100 per cent effective methods of prophylaxis against deep vein thrombosis are available, a reliable screening method is necessary. Even in orthopaedic patients, the ^{125}I-fibrinogen test has been shown to be accurate in detecting thrombi. The high incidence of deep venous thrombosis in patients after myocardial infarction, in patients undergoing prostatectomy and in patients with fractures of the femoral neck has been demonstrated, and some aetiological and prophylactic factors discussed.

REFERENCES

ANTILA, L. E. et al. (1965) *Acta Chir. Scand., Suppl.*, **357**, 95.
BAUER, G. (1940) *Acta Chir. Scand., Suppl.*, **61**, 84.
BECKER, J. et al. (1970) *Acta Radiol. (Diagn.)*, **10**, 513.
BROWDER, F. S. et al. (1959) *Arch. Inst. Cardiol. Mexico*, **29**, 31.
COON, W. W. and COLLER, F. A. (1959) *Surg. Gynec. Obstet.*, **109**, 259.
CULVER, D. et al. (1970) *J. Bone and Jt. Surgery*, **52B**, 61.
EVANS, D. S. and COCKETT, F. B. (1969) *Brit. med. J.*, **2**, 802.
FLANC, C. et al. (1968) *Brit. J. Surg.*, **55**, 742.

FREEARK, J. J. et al. (1967) *Arch. Surg. (Chicago)*, **95**, 566.
FRIEND, J. R. and KAKKAR, V. V. (1970) *J. Obst. Gynaec. Brit. Cwlth*, **77**, 820.
FRIEND, J. R. (1971) Unpublished data.
FRYKHOLM, R. (1939) *Nord. Med.*, **4**, 3534.
HILDEN, T. et al. (1961) *Lancet*, **2**, 327.
KAKKAR, V. V. and FLANC, C. (1968) *Brit. J. Surg.*, **55**, 384.
KAKKAR, V. V. (1969) *Ann. Roy. Coll. Surg. Engl.*, **45**, 257.
KAKKAR, V. V. et al. (1970) *Am. J. Surg.*, **120**, 505.
MAVOR, G. E. and GALLOWAY, J. M. D. (1969) *Brit. J. Surg.*, **56**, 45.
Medical Research Council (1969) Report of the working party on anticoagulant therapy in coronary thrombosis, *Brit. med. J.*, **1**, 335.
MURRAY, T. S. et al. (1970) *Lancet* **2**, 792.
NEGUS, D. et al. (1968) *Brit. J. Surg.*, **55**, 835.
NICOLAIDES, A. N. (1970) Unpublished data.
NICOLAIDES, A. N. et al. (1971) *Brit. med. J.*, **1**, 432.
NICOLAIDES, A. N. et al. (1971) *Brit. J. Radiol.*, **44**, 653.
PINTO, D. J. (1970) *Brit. J. Surg.*, **57**, 349.
SALZMAN, E. W. et al. (1966) *New Engl. J. Med.*, **275**, 122.
SEVITT, S. and GALLAGHER, M. G. (1959) *Lancet*, **2**, 981.
SOLONEN, K. A. (1963) *Acta Orthop. Scand.*, **33**, 329.
STEVEN, J. et al. (1968) *J. Trauma*, **8**, 527.

11 Deep Vein Thrombosis in Obstetric and Gynaecological Patients

J. R. Friend and V. V. Kakkar

INTRODUCTION

Deep vein thrombosis in the lower limb carries a considerable mortality from pulmonary embolism and morbidity from the post-phlebitic syndrome. In obstetrics and gynaecology there has recently been a greater interest in this condition. This is partly due to the widespread use of 'the pill' and the increasing number of operations being carried out on pregnant women. Confinement in this country has become a relatively safe procedure. The maternal mortality surveys from 1961 to 1966 showed that there were some 1,300 maternal deaths in England and Wales in the six-year period, and that the four leading causes of maternal mortality are: abortion, pulmonary embolism, toxaemia and haemorrhage (Table 11.1).

TABLE 11.1

MATERNAL DEATHS IN ENGLAND AND WALES 1961–66

Abortion	272
Pulmonary embolism	224
Toxaemia	171
Haemorrhage	160

The impact of treatment on patients with toxaemia and haemorrhage has steadily reduced their mortality so that pulmonary embolism now stands second only to abortion as a cause of maternal death. The incidence of non-fatal puerperal embolism quoted by various authors varies from 0·27 per cent (Husni et al., 1967; Ullery, 1954) to 1·2 per cent (Bauer, 1946). Similarly the reported incidence of non-fatal thrombo-embolism also shows a wide variation from 4·7 to 1·6 per thousand deliveries (Table 11.2).

These retrospective studies are based on large numbers but all depend on a clinical diagnosis which is known to be unreliable. The ^{125}I-fibrinogen test has been shown to be an accurate method for detecting early and forming thrombi (Atkins and Hawkins, 1965; Flanc et al., 1968; Negus et al., 1968; Kakkar, 1969, 1970). It has also been shown that the test is safe in surgical, orthopaedic and medical patients. However, the test may carry some risk in pregnant women because of the possibility that the radioactive iodine may cross the placenta to reach the foetus; also it may be excreted in the breast milk.

TABLE 11.2

INCIDENCE OF CLINICAL THROMBO-EMBOLISM

	per 1000 *deliveries*
Daniel et al., 1967	4·7
Jeffcoate and Tindall, 1965	3·3
Jeffcoate et al., 1968	2·7
Millar and Robertson, 1968..........	1·6

In this paper we report the results of a study which was designed to investigate these possibilities and to determine the true incidence of this condition in the puerperium and in gynaecological patients.

ANTEPARTUM STUDIES

The problem of deep vein thrombosis during the antenatal period has several important and different aspects compared with other patients at risk. It is difficult to assess the frequency of this condition in antenatal patients because many patients have symptoms in their legs which may not be related to deep vein thrombosis. It is essential to confirm the diagnosis since therapy is essential if deep vein thrombosis exists, and the chances of pulmonary embolism are high. Also the condition that led to the formation of deep vein thrombosis will, almost certainly, remain operative until after the delivery of the conceptus. Thus, the accepted treatment with anticoagulants may have to be continued after confinement, though some carry a considerable risk to the foetus.

The ^{125}I-fibrinogen technique would provide an accurate method of diagnosis and a means of following the progress of the thrombus for at least a week and probably longer. However, the foetus would be subject to the effects of passage of any ^{125}I or ^{125}I-fibrinogen across the placenta. It is obvious that, before a large-scale prospective screening programme with ^{125}I-fibrinogen could be undertaken in this group of patients, the risk of radiation to the foetus should be known accurately. A study was therefore devised in which there were three groups of patients: those who were undergoing hysterotomy for termination of pregnancy and in whom sterilisation was also being performed; those known to have an anencephalic foetus prior to delivery which inevitably would result in still-birth; those who did not breast feed but were willing to express milk for up to one week after delivery.

In the first two groups of patients, following the intravenous injection of 100 mg of sodium iodide to block the thyroid, 100 μci of ^{125}I-fibrinogen were given intravenously prior to operation in the case of hysterotomy or prior to delivery in those patients with an anencephalic foetus. Following delivery of the conceptus, samples of maternal and foetal blood and various foetal tissues were collected for measurement of radioactivity. The results were expressed as a percentage of the maternal whole blood.

RESULTS

The results of this study showed that radioactive iodine tagged to fibrinogen does not enter the foetal circulation but free ^{125}I crosses the placenta and is concentrated in the foetal thyroid. Although the amount of radioactivity to which the foetus is subjected is small, any unnecessary irradiation to a developing foetus is undesirable. These findings clearly indicate that the radioactive fibrinogen test can not be used as routine screening procedure in antepartum patients.

In the remaining group of patients who were expressing breast milk, the ^{125}I-fibrinogen was injected immediately after delivery and daily samples of maternal blood and breast milk were obtained and their radioactive content measured (Fig. 11.1). The amount of radioactivity was expressed as a percentage of the whole blood reading soon after injection.

The results showed that there was a fall in the radioactivity in the blood as the ^{125}I-fibrinogen was metabolised and the free iodine excreted. The radioactivity in the milk, although of a lower magnitude, rose to a maximum around 24 hours and then fell off. These findings show that the radioactive fibringen test is unsuitable for use in lactating mothers.

POST-PARTUM STUDIES

Material for this study consisted of 148 postpartum patients who were staying in hospital for eight days or more and had elected to bottle-feed their babies. In all patients lactation was suppressed with two doses of intramuscular hexoestrol dipropionate (30 mg given within 24 hours of delivery and 15 mg a day later). ^{125}I-labelled fibrinogen (100 μci) was injected intravenously within 8 hours of delivery. One hour prior to this, 100 mg sodium iodide were given intravenously to prevent uptake of ^{125}I by the thyroid gland. Measurement of radioactivity was measured by the procedure described earlier (Kakkar and Howe, page 101).

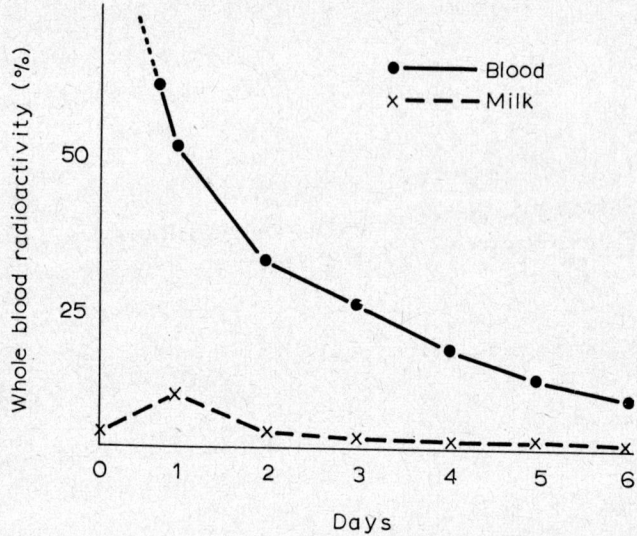

FIG. 11.1. Radioactivity in blood and milk.

RESULTS

In the group of 117 patients who had normal deliveries, three patients developed deep vein thrombosis as detected by the ^{125}I-fibrinogen technique. None was found in the group undergoing Caesarean section (Table 11.3). There was no evidence of pulmonary embolism in any patient.

TABLE 11.3
RESULTS

	Total	Supl. vein thrombosis	Deep vein thrombosis
Vaginal delivery	117	7	3
Caesarean section	31	3	0

The details of the three patients who developed deep vein thrombosis are shown in Table 11.4. In all these cases the diagnosis became apparent at the third postpartum day. The thrombus was confirmed in each case by phlebography, using the technique described by Kakkar and Flanc (1968). In all three patients the thrombosis was confined to the tibial veins. In addition, another six patients developed superficial vein thrombosis.

The present small series gives an incidence of deep vein thrombosis of 3 per cent. However, it should be noted that it is some ten times the quoted incidence of thrombo-embolism in puerperal patients as assessed clinically; in one series the clinical incidence was 0·59 per cent and in another 0·28 per cent (Jeffcoate et al., 1968). It has been shown that patients who have lactation suppressed have a higher incidence of venous thrombosis (Daniel et al., 1967; Jeffcoate et al., 1968). No direct comparison with lactating mothers was

TABLE 11.4

DEEP VEIN THROMBOSES

Patient	Age	Parity	Weight (kgs)	Clinical signs	Obstet. complics.
A	32	0	66	+	—
B	39	4	53·5	—	Bed rest
C	28	3	90	—	P.E.T.

obtained in this trial as there is always some contamination of breast milk by radioactive iodine. Detailed analysis of the three patients who developed deep vein thrombosis revealed some interesting features; the average age of the group of patients studied was 24.4 years of age (range 17–41 years) whereas the ages of the three patients with thrombosis were 28, 32 and 39 years. This agrees with other evidence which associates increasing age with thrombosis (Inman and Vessey, 1968). The parity of two of the three cases was higher than average and two of the patients had been on continued bed rest for some time prior to delivery.

At present, in the absence of effective prophylaxis, the ideal would be to diagnose deep vein thrombosis at the earliest moment in all patients. There is no doubt that treatment is more effective if established at an early stage (Kakkar et al., 1969). If the thrombus is confined to the calf, then the only treatment required is elastic stockings and ambulation. If the thrombus is spreading more proximally into the popliteal and femoral veins, then further treatment should be considered. With such a low incidence of deep vein thrombosis in the puerperium, it would be impractical to use this method of prospective diagnosis in all patients. Its use, however, would be amply justified if a group of patients at risk could be defined. This group might include older women, aged 30 or more, those with a history of previous deep vein thrombosis or pulmonary embolism, those with varicose veins and those who had a traumatic delivery. Work is currently in progress attempting to define such a group. In any patient who develops signs and symptoms suggestive of deep vein thrombosis, this technique can be used as a rapid diagnostic test.

GYNAECOLOGICAL PATIENTS

It is believed that the lithotomy position during operation might increase the risk of deep vein thrombosis, due to the constant pressure on the calf muscles for several hours. Ninety-two patients over the age of 30, undergoing major pelvic surgery either by the abdominal or vaginal route, were investigated. The position of the patient on the operating table was standardised as far as possible. For example, the amount of head-down tilt or the position of attachment of the diathermy pad was always the same. Of these 92 patients, 36 per cent required the lithotomy position with the legs held elevated in stirrups, and 64 per cent were supine with a 5–10° head-down tilt on the table. The technique of the radioactive fibrinogen test used for detecting thrombi in these patients was the same as that described for surgical patients.

RESULTS

The overall incidence of deep vein thrombosis was 17·8 per cent. Of 59 patients who had abdominal operations, 23·7 per cent developed deep vein thrombosis while this complication occurred in only 9 per cent of 33 patients who had vaginal operations (Fig. 11.2).

The incidence is low compared with other prospective postoperative studies using a similar technique; however, the group of patients studied was composed of relatively young females who were not generally ill at the time of operation. Age is believed to be important in relation to the occurrence of thrombosis; although there appears to be an increased incidence over the age of 40 years, the figures from this study do not reach significance. All age groups were affected, 30 per cent of thromboses occurring in patients under 40 years of age. Only one of 17 deep vein thromboses occurred in a patient who had undergone vaginal surgery in the lithotomy position, although 36 per cent of the patients were in this position during operation.

It has been suggested that blood groups A, B and AB have an increased incidence of thrombosis and although there may be a trend in this direction, the numbers in this study were too small to allow a definite conclusion. There was no significant indication that the use of 'the pill', presence of pregnancy or the relationship to the menopause made any difference to the likelihood of developing deep vein thrombosis.

Further analysis of the 13 patients who developed deep vein thrombosis shows that in 10 the thrombus was detected within 72 hours of operation. Symptoms and signs could be elicited in just over half the patients, but their onset was always delayed for at least 24 hours after the initial detection of thrombosis. Nearly half of the patients were entirely asymptomatic throughout.

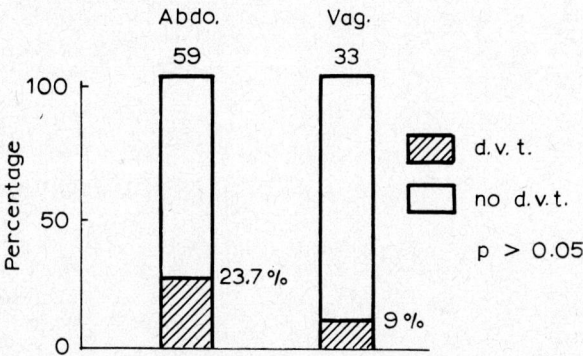

FIG. 11.2. Incidence of deep venous thrombosis.

Over half of the patients had ascending phlebograms of the affected limb and in all cases the thrombus was confirmed. The extent of the thrombus correlated well with the distribution as mapped out by the radioactive fibrinogen test. Soleal and tibial veins were the site of the majority of thromboses and in all but one of the patients there was no involvement of the popliteal, femoral or iliac veins.

In six patients the lesions were bilateral and in all these cases the time of onset and extent of development of thrombus in both legs was similar. Of the remaining eight cases, six occurred in the left calf and two in the right calf.

SUMMARY

The trans-placental passage of free ^{125}I and its appearance in milk contraindicate use of the ^{125}I-fibrinogen test during pregnancy and in mothers who breast-feed.

The incidence of post-partum deep venous thrombosis, diagnosed by this test was 3 per cent. In gynaecological patients, there was a higher incidence of venous thrombosis in patients undergoing an abdominal operation (24 per cent) compared with a vaginal operation (9 per cent). The lithotomy position was not associated with a high incidence.

REFERENCES

ATKINS, P. and HAWKINS, L. A. (1965) *Lancet*, **2,** 1217.
BAUER, G. (1946) *Lancet*, **1,** 447.
DANIEL, D. G. et al. (1967) *Lancet*, **2,** 287.
FLANC, C. et al. (1968) *Brit. J. Surg.*, **55,** 742.
HUSNI, E. A. et al. (1967) *Amer. J. Obst. Gynec.*, **97,** 901.
INMAN, W. H. W. and VESSEY, M. P. (1968) *Brit. med. J.*, **2,** 193.
JEFFCOATE, F. N. A. et al. (1968) *Brit. med. J.*, **4,** 19.
KAKKAR, V. V. and FLANC, C. (1968) *Brit. J. Surg.*, **55,** 384.
KAKKAR, V. V. et al. (1969) *Brit. med. J.*, **1,** 806.
KAKKAR, V. V. et al. (1970) *Lancet*, **1,** 540.
ULLERY, J. C. (1954) *Amer. J. Obst. Gynec.*, **68,** 1243.

12 Discussion

Negus: Mr. Cotton has suggested that our work (Browse and Negus, 1970) on galvanic stimulation of the legs has many drawbacks. This technique gave similar results; there are no problems provided one has a trained technician and suitable electrodes. We produced no burns.

Doran: We too have used this method on several hundred patients, including two clinical trials of 200 patients each, and have had no burns.

Hicks: It is generally agreed that the most important function of detecting venous thrombosis is to reduce the morbidity and mortality from pulmonary embolism. Is there any evidence that site, extent or time course of thrombosis affects the morbidity from pulmonary embolism? Do clinical or more elegant diagnostic criteria offer a means of predicting which patients are at risk?

Kakkar: As yet, the number of patients studied is too small to be certain which patients with a positive radioactive fibrinogen test will subsequently die from pulmonary embolism.

This technique enables one to detect thrombi, follow their course and identify the group of patients likely to develop pulmonary embolism. We have shown quite convincingly that, if a thrombus has extended above the knee, pulmonary embolism is likely. However, out of this small group of patients, none died from pulmonary embolism.

Sigel: I entirely agree that the complications—pulmonary embolism, whether non-fatal or fatal, and the post-phlebitic syndrome are the best endpoints in judging any technique in the detection of venous thrombosis. We are currently planning a study which will utilize risk factor analysis to determine the best predictors of pulmonary embolism. Two factors which we shall consider will be clinical evaluation and ultrasound detection of thrombosis. Our preliminary estimate is that we will need about 8000 patients in order to see sufficient complications for this analysis.

Wessler: Is it possible to get adequate venographic visualisation of the iliac veins from an injection in the foot? Secondly, is there agreement that thrombosis in the iliac veins occurs by proximal progression, or may it occur independently?

Kakkar: The iliac veins can almost always be demonstrated by filling the veins selectively, using an image intensifier to follow the contrast medium.

Widmer: Our experience involving about 150 patients with deep vein thrombosis, demonstrated phlebographically, confirms Mr. Kakkar's results. The external and common iliac, but not the internal iliac vein, are readily visualised, unless the femoral is closed—a situation which prevails in about 10 per cent of cases.

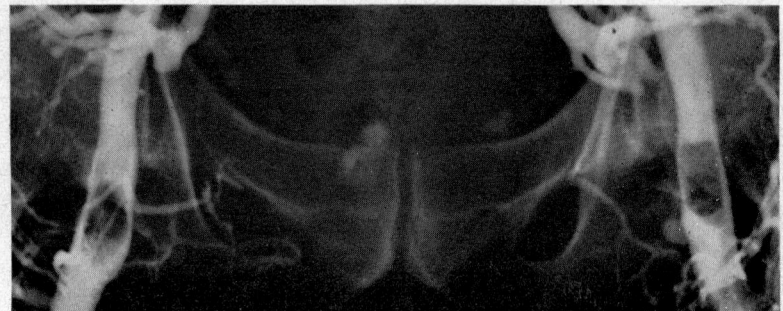

Fig. 12.1. Primary iliofemoral thrombi.

Negus: While agreeing with Mr. Kakkar that most venous thromboses arise in the calf and of these some propagate along the femoral vein, there is a small but dangerous minority of deep vein thromboses which arise per primam in the upper femoral or iliac veins. These are not infrequently seen in phlebograms (Fig. 12.1). These thrombi, although a small minority of the whole problem, are potentially dangerous and in this situation they cannot be detected by the ^{125}I-fibrinogen technique. It is therefore urged that this technique should be accompanied by other methods of investigation, either phlebography or Doppler Ultrasound.

Sasahara: I believe that this symposium on thromboembolism would be incomplete without some mention of impedance plethysmography for the detection of deep venous thrombosis. Although the method is not new, its adaptation for the venous system by Dr. H. B. Wheeler, Chief of Surgery at our Hospital (V.A. Hospital, West Roxbury, Massachusetts) is new. As the newest and least invasive of all the

DISCUSSION

diagnostic methods discussed today, its use is based upon the changing blood volume of the limbs with respiration, and Ohm's Law. Since blood is an excellent conductor of electricity, the resistance or impedance of a given amount of current which passes between two points is inversely proportional to the blood volume contained between the two points. Thus, in inspiration, limb venous return is diminished, limb blood volume is increased and the impedance of a known amount of current is diminished. In expiration, limb venous return is augmented, limb blood volume is diminished and the

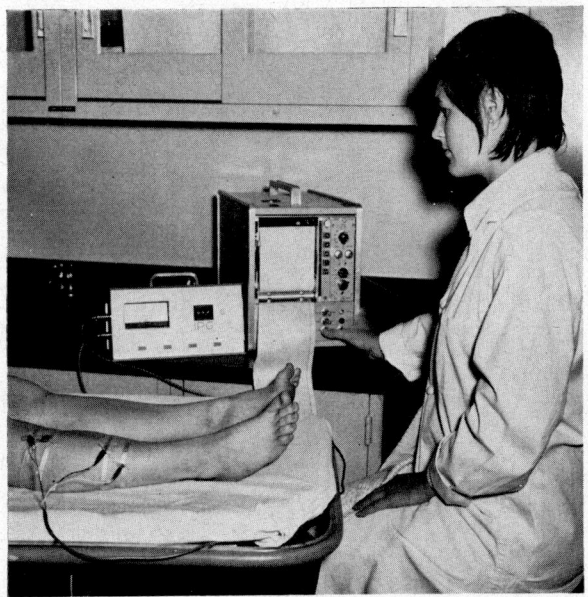

Fig. 12.2. Use of a direct-writer in recording fluctuations in impedance with respiration.

impedance increases. The fluctuations in impedance with respiration may be recorded with a direct-writer (Fig. 12.2). When deep venous thrombosis is present, little variation occurs in limb blood volume, and hence in impedance. The resulting tracing is a flattened curve, as illustrated in the bottom tracing (left calf) of Fig. 12.3. The black horizontal bar represents inspiration and the rise in the curve (upper tracing) indicates decreasing impedance.

There has been unbelievably good correlation with venography in the detection of deep venous thrombosis. In legs which were symptomatic but negative by venography, the impedance plethysmograph has been normal. Some 700 patients have been studied to

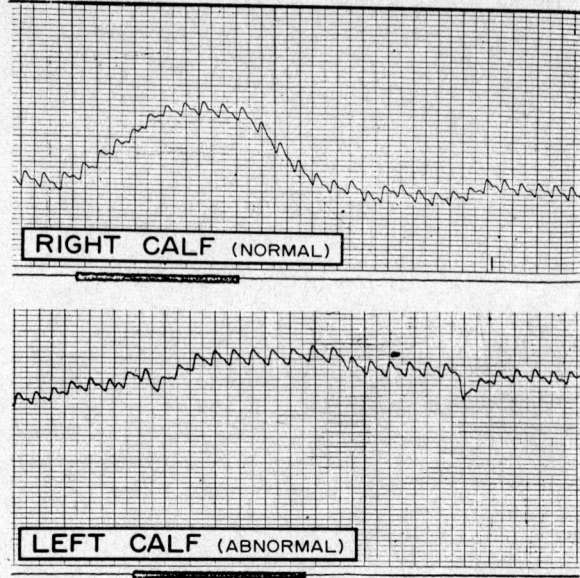

Fig. 12.3. Normal and abnormal impedance tracings.

date and the data have been published in *Surgery* (1971) 70, 20–26. The changes in impedance may also be quantified and in certain conditions such as deep vein thrombosis with collateral formation, there is a qualitative change as well. Although the method has yet to be compared with the radioactive fibrinogen technique for sensitivity, current data indicate that this is a most promising and sensitive screening tool for deep venous thrombosis.

REFERENCES

Browse, N. L. and Negus, D. (1970) *Brit. med. J.*, **3,** 615.

PART III
MEDICAL TREATMENT

13 Is Thrombolytic Therapy Justified?
S. Sherry

Experience with the commonly available anticoagulants, heparin and the coumarins, has provided us with a fairly clear picture of their usefulness and limitations. In general, these agents have been proven to be of value for:

Prevention of venous thrombotic disease.
Inhibition of thrombus growth and subsequent embolisation, whether venous or arterial.
On the other hand, they appear to be of relatively little value for:
Prevention of arterial thrombosis.
Resolution of an established thrombus, whether arterial or venous.

Since thrombolytic therapy is primarily designed for rapid thrombus resolution, the first question to be posed is whether there is justification for developing therapeutic modes for inducing rapid thrombus resolution. The answer is *an unqualified yes*. The potential benefits to be achieved from the rapid resolution of the circulatory obstruction produced by a thromboembolism includes a decrease in mortality from such episodes, diminished morbidity arising from acute thromboembolic events, and the prevention of chronic disability arising from the consequences of an impaired circulation.

The next question to be posed is whether there is a need to develop a medical thrombo-embolectomy when surgical procedures are already available and continually improving. The answer again is *an unqualified yes*. While surgical procedures will always have more flexibility in that, besides thrombo-embolectomy, other obstructing lesions can be removed and, where indicated, by-passes and other forms of reconstructive procedures can be undertaken, thrombolytic therapy can be instituted more quickly; it is potentially available for use by all physicians; and it can be administered for lesions currently inaccessable to most surgeons and in patients critically ill and not likely to tolerate surgery well. This is not to imply that thrombolytic therapy will replace surgery in the management of acute occlusive vascular lesions, but that it may well have advantages in the treatment of certain patients, either when used alone or in conjunction with surgery.

Before answering the key question, i.e., as to whether current forms of thrombolytic therapy are justified, let us consider whether the sequential steps necessary for the appropriate development of such a therapy have been met. At the present time two powerful clot dissolving agents have been available for pharmacologic study, clinical investigation and therapeutic evaluation. When used in appropriate dosage both agents have been shown to induce and sustain an active thrombolytic state in the patient's circulating blood which is readily demonstrable and easily reproducible within reasonable limits. Furthermore this induced state has been shown to be associated with the dissolution of thromboemboli in vivo. In addition, the hazards involved in this pharmacological state have been well documented, as have the other aspects of toxicity. Thus justification of these agents for therapeutic purposes now depends primarily on documentation of clinical benefit, and that such benefit outweighs the risks involved in their use. What then has been the clinical experience with each of these agents?

STREPTOKINASE

The experience with streptokinase already has assumed extensive proportions, sufficient in size and scope to indicate the areas where it is likely to prove beneficial. Streptokinase is a secretory protein of haemolytic streptococci and the most widely used laboratory activator of human plasminogen, the naturally occurring fibrinolytic enzyme precursor. It was originally developed for thrombolytic purposes in the United States where it served as a model for establishing the scientific basis and therapeutic potential for the in vivo use of plasminogen activators. The investigation of streptokinase was terminated in the States in 1960 because of its antigenicity and the tendency for preparations to elicit undesirable and ill-understood pyrogenic reactions. Since the substance could be produced relatively inexpensively and in large quantities, several European pharmaceutical firms undertook the further development of streptokinase and it subsequently became commercially available on the Continent. Pyrogenicity was minimised by the production of more purified preparations, and therapy was streamlined through the introduction of practical dosage schedules which, when monitored by simple laboratory tests, circumvented many of the difficulties encountered earlier. Although the antigenicity of streptokinase will always impose restrictions on its utility, particularly in the retreatment of individuals suffering from recurrent thrombotic episodes, this has not proven to be a deterrent to its clinical acceptance. It is estimated that perhaps fifty thousand patients have received streptokinase therapy; most of the experience has been in West Germany, Switzerland, Sweden, Belgium, Australia and Great Britain, and indications exist that streptokinase is being used in Russia as well. Currently, streptokinase is, once again, under active study in the United States.

The use of plasminogen activators, like streptokinase, is based on data which suggest that the most sensitive mechanism for thrombolysis involves the diffusion of an activator into the thrombus with conversion of the plasminogen within the thrombus to the active fibrin dissolving enzyme, plasmin; thus, one of the practical therapeutic questions has been whether local perfusion of an occluded vessel with streptokinase would have advantages over the systemic intravenous administration of the agent. Though this question is not resolved, most investigators agree that systemic intravenous administration probably achieves as good a result as local perfusion; thus unless a catheter is already in situ, no striking benefit is likely to accrue from such an ancillary procedure.

Most investigators are now using a fixed dosage schedule, i.e., a loading dose of 250,000 units of streptokinase followed by a sustaining infusion of 100,000 units per hour. While patients vary greatly in their resistance to streptokinase, due to the presence of variable amounts of antistreptokinase and other inhibitory substances, this regimen contains sufficient streptokinase to overcome the resistance of approximately 85–90 per cent of the patient population and maintain free circulating levels of the agent sufficient to induce and sustain an active thrombolytic state. While the latter can be monitored by measurements of circulating fibrinolytic activity, the only test necessary is the thrombin time, i.e., the speed of clotting upon the addition of an excess of thrombin to plasma. In the presence of thrombolytic agents, the thrombin time reflects the appearance and accumulation of fibrinogen break-down products, and indirectly becomes a measure of the activity of the thrombolytic state. Thus, in patients with high resistance, the thrombin time shows little change, suggesting the need for a higher dose; alternatively, an excessive increase in the thrombin time indicates high levels of circulating proteolytic activity and an enhanced risk of bleeding, and may call for a decrease in the dose level.

The major hazard with streptokinase, as with other thrombolytic agents, is bleeding; this is most often encountered at the scene of invasive procedures (venous cut-downs, venepunctures, arterial punctures, etc.) or at the site of intramuscular injections. Bleeding from these sites is usually controllable by local pressure but on occasion more serious bleeding may occur spontaneously or into areas of trauma or recent operative wounds. The contraindications for streptokinase are the same as for anticoagulants. Other undesirable effects attributable to streptokinase are an occasional severe pyrogenic reaction, rash and, in rare instances, an anaphylactoid-like syndrome.

While investigators have been concerned over the possibility that dissolving clots may embolise, this has not proven to be a significant hazard; thrombi undergoing dissolution appear to shrink progressively in size rather than break up into fragments. The question also has been raised as to whether a prolonged thrombolytic state may be followed by a 'rebound' thrombotic state at sites other than the original lesion. Short courses of streptokinase therapy, i.e., for twenty-four hours, when followed by adequate anticoagulation, have not been associated with unexpected thrombotic events. With longer courses of therapy, new thrombi occasionally have been observed even in the presence of anticoagulation; however the significance of these casual observations requires further clarification.

DEEP VENOUS THROMBOSIS

Clinical experience with streptokinase covers almost all types of thromboembolic disease, certain areas having been studied more adequately than others. The observations on acute deep vein thrombosis indicate that about 50–60 per cent of the treated vessels will show considerable angiographic clearing after streptokinase therapy, and the chance of resolution is much higher if the streptokinase is given within 96 hours of the clinical onset of symptoms. When sufficient evidence is provided that thrombus dissolution decreases the incidence of post-phlebitic venous insufficiency, then thrombolytic therapy may well become the initiating treatment for the management of deep vein thrombosis.

ARTERIAL THROMBOEMBOLISM

In acute arterial thrombosis involving the lower extremities, satisfactory dissolution of thrombi can be anticipated in approximately half the treated patients; in embolic disease, the incidence of success is much higher. Surgery is still preferred to fibrinolytic therapy for aorto-iliac occlusion since the results of endarterectomy for this lesion are generally excellent, but streptokinase is considered by many as more efficacious than surgery for the management of occlusions situated in the popliteal artery or more distally. In femoral artery thrombosis, streptokinase yields results comparable to surgery and currently is being used first in a number of centres unless there is evidence to suggest irreversible damage to the limb.

Opinions differ on the use of streptokinase for the management of chronic arterial occlusions of the lower extremity: some claim it is quite useful while others are less enthusiastic.

PULMONARY EMBOLISM

In acute pulmonary embolism, 24 hours of streptokinase therapy has produced an effect similar to that recently reported for urokinase; significant lysis of pulmonary emboli has been achieved with a restoration of haemodynamic abnormalities toward normal. As with urokinase, the effects are more striking with massive pulmonary embolism than with involvement of the smaller pulmonary arteries; this is not an unexpected finding since emboli in the main pulmonary artery or its major branches are more exposed to the action of the clot-dissolving agent. When one considers the high mortality associated with pulmonary embolectomy, particularly in the aged and in those with underlying heart disease, it is likely that thrombolytic therapy will become the initial therapy of choice for the management of most patients seriously ill with an acute massive pulmonary embolism. In this regard, the experience of Miller *et al.* (1971) with streptokinase in acute pulmonary embolism is of considerable interest, and is consistent with the general observation that, in centres where thrombolytic therapy is used, the numbers of patients coming to pulmonary embolectomy has been reduced significantly.

MYOCARDIAL INFARCTION

A major goal for thrombolytic therapy, from the very inception of its development, was to determine its usefulness in the management of acute myocardial infarction. Anticoagulant therapy as presently practiced, is not designed to have a striking impact on the morbidity and mortality from acute myocardial infarction; its value in this disorder is restricted to thrombus growth in the coronary vessels, and to the prevention of venous thrombosis, pulmonary embolism, mural thrombus formation and systemic embolisation. The former does not appear to be an important consideration, while the latter complications account for approximately 6 per cent of the deaths. Intensive anticoagulant therapy probably has eliminated half of these or more but such a gain represents only a small fraction of the problem of survival following an acute infarct.

Pump failure is the most important consideration, and more appropriate for its treatment would be the rapid restoration of blood flow, through removal of the occluding thrombus. If the latter can be achieved medically by thrombolytic agents, in a simple and reliable manner without undue hazard, the following potential benefits might be obtained:

1. Improved cardiac output resulting from the salvage of some of the dying but reclaimable muscle, the augmentation of myocardial function in areas of marginal ischaemia and the prevention of recurrent or extending infarctions.
2. A decrease in disabling or fatal arrhythmias from relief of the irritability arising from the marginal zone of ischaemia.
3. Avoidance of some of the thromboembolic complications through the lysis of incipient thrombi forming on the damaged endocardium and in peripheral veins at sites of stasis.

The experience with streptokinase in acute myocardial infarction already has assumed significant proportions with four major trials having been undertaken in patients diagnosed as having this disease. Two are German trials involving the same group of hospitals; the first was concluded in 1966, the other in 1970. A third study involving 8 hospitals in Belgium, Holland, Germany and Austria and referred to as the European Working Party Trial also was concluded in 1970, while the fourth is an Australian investigation still in progress.

In all these trials, the controls received conventional anticoagulant therapy, while the streptokinase group received the thrombolytic agent for 24 hours, beginning on the first day of their infarction, and then were followed on anticoagulant therapy. The streptokinase was given in a small volume through a sustaining intravenous infusion employing a fixed dose schedule, usually a loading dose of 250,000 units followed by 100,000 units per hour; this induced and maintained a striking clot dissolving state in approximately 90 per cent of the patients.

The first trial (Schmutzler *et al.*, 1966), conducted in Germany included 558 patients, of whom 297 were treated with streptokinase and 261 with anticoagulants. The early mortality, late mortality and total mortality was considerably reduced in the streptokinase group; the difference in the total mortality, i.e. 17 per cent for the streptokinase group as compared to 27 per cent in the controls, was significant at a p value of 0·05. Other conclusions drawn from this study were: streptokinase therapy reduced mortality between the second and fortieth day after infarction from 21·7 to 14·1 per cent; no significant risk could be attributed to the use of streptokinase in acute myocardial infarction; serial differences in the electrocardiogram between the two groups suggested that streptokinase was beneficial in myocardial infarction; and finally the higher incidence of rudimentary infarction in patients treated with streptokinase suggested that, in a number of patients, the early use of thrombolytic therapy was reducing the extent of cardiac muscle necrosis. Since the first trial did not employ appropriate randomisation, corrections were made in the second German trial recently concluded (Schmutzler *et al.*, 1970). The data from the latter, while still unpublished, also shows a significant mortality difference among the 245 patients studied, and supports the observations made in the first trial, i.e., streptokinase treatment reduces the mortality from acute myocardial infarction by approximately 30-35 per cent.

The most extensive study to date is the European Working Party's Trial which was coordinated by Verstraete in Louvain and published in 1971. In this study, there were 163 deaths in the 730 patients observed over a 30 day period—an average mortality of 22·3 per cent. In the streptokinase group of 373 patients, 69 died—a mortality of 18·5 per cent; while in the heparin group (i.e. heparin for the first 24 hours followed by coumarin therapy), there were 94 deaths in 357 patients at risk—a mortality of 26·3 per cent. The difference in mortality was significant at the 1 per cent level and represents a total reduction in mortality by streptokinase of 30 per cent. While there were minor differences in the pattern of deaths among the two groups, the major and only significant feature was in the incidence of heart failure as a cause of death; 16 of the patients treated with streptokinase died as a result of a failing myocardium, while 38, or more than twice as many, on anticoagulant therapy alone died as a result of this disorder. This difference was significant at the 0·001 level.

An increased number of complications was seen during streptokinase therapy as compared to heparin in this trial, but this was due almost exclusively to more patients on streptokinase showing a temperature rise of more than 1°C and to a higher frequency of bleeding at puncture sites. Haematomata at other sites, macroscopic haematuria and melaena occurred equally but rarely in both treatment groups. The treatment was interrupted because of bleeding in 6 streptokinase-treated patients and 2 heparin-treated patients; in only 1 patient was transfusion necessary and this patient was receiving heparin.

As for complications appearing during the subsequent follow up period, i.e., from the 2nd to 30th day following the initial streptokinase or heparin therapy, shock was observed less frequently in the streptokinase-treated patients but the numbers were too small to be of significance. However a significant difference, i.e., with a p value of less than 0·05, was observed for reinfarction; this complication appeared less frequently following streptokinase.

Autopsy reports were available on 42 streptokinase-treated and 49 heparin-treated patients. Heart rupture occurred in 10 streptokinase and 14 heparin patients, and cerebral bleeding occurred in 2 patients of each group; thus generalised or local bleeding into the brain or heart was not found to be a prevalent cause of death with this form of streptokinase therapy.

Finally, in the fourth study still underway in Australia (Hale, 1970) the published information on the first 127 cases, i.e., 64 streptokinase-treated and 63 heparin-treated, again suggests a trend towards a difference in mortality: 9·4 per cent for streptokinase and 14·3 per cent for heparin, i.e., a reduction in mortality in the streptokinase group of 34 per cent.

Thus, observations on the use of streptokinase in acute myocardial infarction may be summarised as follows: 4 separate trials involving a total of almost 1700 patients seem to confirm each other and suggest that streptokinase therapy reduces mortality in acute myocardial infarction by approximately 30–35 per cent; furthermore most of the potential benefits of this treatment, previously described as theoretical, have been confirmed by clinical study.

UROKINASE

The experience with urokinase is limited, since the material has never been commercially available and its investigation is being restricted to carefully controlled trials in specific lesions. Urokinase is a plasminogen activator normally present in human urine; it is made by the kidneys presumably to keep the renal tubules and urinary tract free from fibrinous deposits. Its virtues lie in its non-antigenicity, non-pyrogenicity or other toxicity except bleeding, and its ability to induce a more reliable thrombolytic state with milder aberrations in the haemostatic mechanism than are seen with streptokinase. After overcoming production problems, partially purified preparations of human urokinase, free of toxic impurities, were prepared by two major American pharmaceutical firms, and the clinical investigation of the agent was sponsored by the National Heart and Lung Institute in the United States.

Following the acquisition of appropriate pharmacological data in man, the initial evaluation of urokinase was undertaken in acute pulmonary embolism; most important in this choice was that pulmonary angiography, haemodynamic measurements and lung scanning were available to assess the effects of this agent on the embolism.

The recently concluded first phase of the multi-institutional Urokinase-Pulmonary Embolism Trial reported in 1970 and described in these proceedings by Dr. Sasahara (p. 195) has established the ability of urokinase to lyse pulmonary emboli, increase pulmonary capillary perfusion and improve the haemodynamic abnormalities associated with the disorder. While these observations have important therapeutic implications, particularly for patients with massive pulmonary embolism and shock, the trial evaluated only one urokinase treatment regimen, i.e., a 12 hour infusion. Accordingly, while thrombus resolution was unequivocal, nevertheless it was not dramatic in terms of lysing the entire pulmonary occlusion or of completely resolving the haemodynamic abnormalities. On the basis of experience, it may be predicted that a longer treatment period will more closely approach the goal of a complete medical thrombectomy without further increasing the risk of a haemorrhage; certainly if this can be accomplished it would be a much more useful regimen for the treatment of patients critically ill with acute pulmonary embolism, as well as for the management of other thromboembolic lesions. For this reason the second phase, which is referred to as the Urokinase-Streptokinase Pulmonary Embolism Trial, is underway; patients are now being randomised into three groups: those receiving 12 hours of urokinase as before; those receiving a 24 hour infusion of urokinase and those receiving 24 hours of streptokinase therapy. Besides yielding information as to the effects of a longer urokinase infusion, this new phase will provide the first comparison between the thrombolytic effects and hazards of the two major promising thrombolytic agents when used according to current dosage schedules. Phase II was initiated at the end of 1970 and over 80 patients have been studied to date; hopefully this phase will be concluded relatively quickly and yield information most helpful in the planning and conduct of a major National Heart and Lung Institute sponsored trial aimed at evaluating the benefits, if any, of urokinase and streptokinase on the mortality and morbidity of acute myocardial infarction.

Mention also should be made of the urokinase myocardial infarction trial now underway and involving medical centres in several European countries, which is being coordinated in Basel. This trial has been in progress for close to 2 years, and while it is known that several hundred patients have been entered into the trial, no results are available as yet.

CONCLUSION

Now, to return to the key question posed in this presentation, i.e., is thrombolytic therapy justified? The answer is *a qualified yes!* The therapy is capable of achieving significant thrombolysis in vivo but with a real risk of bleeding. At present many of the clinical benefits appear to outweigh the risks for certain lesions, but not for others. A more extensive experience with carefully controlled trials is still needed to delineate better the indications, contraindications, clinical accomplishments and hazards. Only when sufficient data is at hand can a final judgement be made. However, it should be recognised that thrombolytic therapy is in its infancy; under the circumstances and considering its potential, ample justification exists for the active encouragement and further development of thrombolytic therapy. Relative to this latter point, a real need exists for studies aimed at improving our present regimens so as to increase the rate and extent of lysis without increasing the risk of bleeding or, alternatively, to reduce the bleeding hazard without sacrificing the lytic effects of therapy.

REFERENCES

EUROPEAN WORKING PARTY (1971) *Brit. med. J.*, **3,** 325.
HALE, G. S. (1970) *Aust. Ann. Med.*, Suppl. 1, **19,** 63.
MILLER, G. A. H. *et al.* (1971) *Brit. med. J.*, **2,** 681.
SCHMUTZLER, R. *et al.* (1966) *Deutsche Med. Wschr.*, **91,** 581.
SCHMUTZLER, R. *et al.* (1970) *XIII International Congress of Haematology.* Munich, August 2–8, 1970.
UROKINASE PULMONARY EMBOLISM TRIAL STUDY GROUP (1970) *J.A.M.A.*, **214,** 2163.

14 Drug Therapy of Venous Thromboembolism
D. P. Thomas

INTRODUCTION

The medical treatment of venous thrombosis and pulmonary embolism is based primarily on the selective use of various potent drugs. Some of these agents have been studied for many years, and their therapeutic role is clearly defined; other drugs have so far received only limited clinical trial and their potential contribution is still uncertain. At present, several new drugs are undergoing clinical trial, or old drugs are being studied in new ways, for the prophylaxis and treatment of venous thromboembolism. A period of stability in the methods of treatment is now being challenged by the claims of new drugs. It seems logical to insist, however, that a new drug must be significantly superior, whether it be more effective, safer, easier to administer and control, or cheaper, if it is to replace accepted therapy. In this paper, the main categories of drugs employed in the prophylaxis and treatment of thromboembolic disease will be considered, and their relative contribution in the management of the disease critically assessed. Attention will be confined to those drugs which have a direct action on the disease process, for example, anticoagulants, and no account will be given of other drugs, such as digitalis, which may be used in the overall management of the patient.

PROPHYLAXIS

ANTICOAGULANT DRUGS

The modern era of anticoagulant prophylaxis of venous thromboembolism dates from 1959, when Sevitt and Gallagher published their classic controlled trial on patients with fractured necks of femur. Three hundred patients were separated equally into control and treated groups. Treated patients were placed on oral anticoagulant drugs on admission to the hospital, and an operation was usually performed the next day. This was a clinical-pathological study, in which virtually everybody who died came to autopsy; because it was an elderly population, there was a high death rate. Complete dissections were performed, including the leg veins. The incidence of thrombosis at autopsy fell from 29 out of 35 to 3 out of 21. In fact, in these three patients, treatment had been stopped. Embolism caused or contributed significantly to death in 15 control patients as compared to 2 in the treated group. Sevitt demonstrated in this and subsequent studies that, provided the prothrombin time, using a human brain thromboplastin, is kept above twice the control level, significant venous thrombosis is not observed at autopsy (Hume et al., 1970).

There is now considerable evidence as to the benefits of anti-coagulant prophylaxis in high-risk patients, and the efficacy of this form of prophylaxis, if properly carried out and carefully monitored, can be regarded as established. Orthopaedic surgeons have perhaps been among the most enthusiastic supporters of the value of prophylactic anticoagulant therapy (Harris et al., 1967). For example, in over 1000 consecutive patients undergoing elective mold arthroplasty of the hip at the Massachusetts General Hospital, treated with prophylactic anticoagulant therapy, only 6 pulmonary emboli were clinically evident, and none was fatal (Harris, 1971). A fatality rate from pulmonary embolism of 1–2 per cent would be expected in such patients not receiving prophylactic therapy. While the benefits of prophylactic anticoagulant therapy are seen most clearly in patients with fractured hips and following elective hip surgery, there is no reason to believe the benefits are confined to orthopaedic patients. It is arguable that all patients over the age of 40 who will be confined to bed for a week or more because of trauma or an operation should be treated with anticoagulants unless a contraindication exists. Equally, there are many medical patients, such as those with congestive heart failure, in whom prophylactic anticoagulant therapy should be employed more readily. While the risk of haemorrhage is real, it is acceptably low if proper precautions are taken. Most important of all is the recognition that the hazards of treatment are substantially less than the dangers of thromboembolic disease. One of the most noticeable features of anticoagulant therapy is that many physicians are reluctant to employ such treatment, even in high-risk patients. While the search for safer and better drugs must continue, it is well to remember that venous thrombosis is already basically a preventable disease. It is not so much the absence of effective drugs, but the frequent reluctance to use them which characterises the treatment of this disease.

DEXTRAN

Concurrent trials by several workers, especially in Sweden, have shown that dextran (usually dextran-70) reduces the incidence of thromboembolism among general surgical cases, in patients with fractured necks of femur, and in gynaecological subjects undergoing surgery. Bygdeman *et al.* (1970) listed 8 surgical studies in which a total of 1321 patients had been given dextran-70 prophylactically, and compared them with a similar number who were controls. Seemingly, there was something like a four-fold reduction in fatal emboli in the dextran-treated patients. However, in 6 of these 8 studies, there was no significant difference between control and

TABLE 14.1

A COMPARISON OF THE EFFECT OF DEXTRAN AND AN ORAL ANTICOAGULANT ON THE INCIDENCE OF VENOUS THROMBOSIS IN THE LEGS (%)

Study	Diagnostic technique	Incidence of venous thrombosis		Significance
		Dextran	Anticoagulant	
Lambie et al. 1970	^{125}I-fibrinogen	10	30	$P < 0.01$
Salzman et al. 1971	Clinical	10	9	N.S.
Bronge et al. 1971	Phlebography	42	34	N.S.

treated patients in the incidence of fatal emboli. Caution is required in accepting a statistically significant difference that may be present in the aggregate, but which is absent in the individual trial. To emphasise this point, a recent prospective, double-blind, randomly allocated study at Johns Hopkins Hospital found that the prophylactic administration of dextran-70 to high-risk surgical patients reduced neither the incidence of pulmonary emboli nor the overall mortality rate (Brisman *et al.*, 1971).

Three recent studies have compared prophylaxis with dextran and oral anticoagulant drugs (Table 14.1).

In one study using a labelled fibrinogen test for diagnosis, warfarin begun on the 2nd post-operative day was compared with dextran-70 during and after gynaecological surgery. (Lambie *et al.*, 1970). Salzman and colleagues compared warfarin begun on the evening after operation with dextran-40, and used clinical criteria for diagnosing thromboembolism (Salzman *et al.*, 1971). Bronge and colleagues (1971) compared the effect of dicumarol and dextran-70 in patients with femoral neck fractures, and diagnosed venous thrombosis by phlebography 3 weeks after the accident. Two out of the three studies found no significant difference between dextran and an anticoagulant drug, although in the one study both protected the patients and in the other study neither seemed to! (Table I). In all 3 studies, the anticoagulant drug was given after operation, when the criticism could be made that it was already too late to achieve effective prophylaxis. The claim that dextran-70 protected against venous thrombosis as diagnosed by labelled fibrinogen has not been confirmed by Kakkar (1972), who failed to find a protective effect post-operatively with dextran-70.

In 169 patients who underwent vitallium mold arthroplasty of the hip, no significant difference was observed in the incidence of thromboembolic complications between the warfarin, aspirin, and dextran-treated groups (Salzman *et al.*, 1971). However, all 3 groups were significantly different from a previous untreated control group, whereas the fourth group, given dipyridamole, was not. A most interesting observation that emerged from this study was the finding that bleeding complications did not differ significantly between the 4 groups.

The advantages claimed for dextran prophylaxis are the absence of bleeding complications and the lack of the need for laboratory control of therapy compared to oral anticoagulant drugs; but the disadvantages are the need for intravenous administration and the possibility of overloading the circulation, especially among those with limited cardiopulmonary reserves. However, many questions remain to be answered. If dextran reduces the accumulation of radioactive counts in the legs immediately after operation, as Lambie and colleagues have claimed with the labelled fibrinogen test, does it therefore follow that there is a reduced incidence of venous thrombosis 3 weeks later, when looked for on phlebography? Bronge *et al.* pointed out that phlebography at 3 weeks (at which time they failed to demonstrate a protective effect of dextran) is not the same thing as phlebography performed 2–10 months after the events, which is when some of the other Swedish dextran studies looked for venous thrombosis.

ASPIRIN

Salzman *et al.* (1971) studied the protection against venous thrombosis and pulmonary embolism afforded by 3 drugs affecting platelet function in a controlled study of patients undergoing surgery of the hip. Prophylactic administration of dipyridamole, aspirin and dextran-40 was compared with the effects of warfarin, and it was claimed that the results with aspirin were better than those in an untreated group previously reported. However, while the incidence of venous thrombosis as detected by ordinary clinical criteria was lower in the patients taking aspirin—as compared to the previous controlled group—the incidence of pulmonary embolism was not reduced. This paradoxical result raises the question of whether the administration of aspirin (1·2 grams daily) may have masked some of the clinical diagnostic criteria for venous thrombosis in the legs, such as pain, tenderness and increased temperature. Recent evidence that aspirin prevents the synthesis of prostaglandins (Vane, 1971), and also prevents the release of prostaglandins from platelets by thrombin (Smith and Willis, 1971) may well be relevant. There is increasing evidence that prostaglandins are mediators of the inflammatory response, and it is possible that platelet prostaglandins contribute to the symptoms of pain, tenderness and increased temperature evoked by a thrombus in the leg veins. This would explain the *apparent* success of aspirin in preventing venous thrombosis, and its lack of success in preventing pulmonary emboli. This consideration also receives support from the results of a Medical Research Council study on the effects of high and low dosage aspirin in preventing ^{125}I-fibrinogen detected post-operative venous thrombosis. Preliminary reports from this study suggests that neither low doses (0·6 g) nor high doses (2·4 g) of daily aspirin prevent venous thrombosis as detected by this highly sensitive technique. In 58 patients, O'Brien *et al.* (1971) found no difference in the incidence of thrombosis in patients receiving no aspirin, low-dose aspirin or high-dose aspirin. Thus, while aspirin may mask some of the clinical symptoms of venous thrombosis, there is no evidence that it reduces either the incidence of pulmonary embolism or the incidence of venous thrombosis as detected by the labelled fibrinogen technique.

The use of aspirin, or indeed any platelet-active drug, may also be questioned on theoretical grounds. While aspirin is highly effective in preventing a collagen-platelet interaction in vitro, whether such a process is an essential step in the pathogenesis of *venous* thrombosis is problematical. Incipient thrombi are found in the valve pockets of human leg veins; they are usually of mixed platelet and fibrin composition, and there is no microscopical evidence that they result from overt endothelial damage. However, there may be some subtle damage to the endothelium in the valve pockets, leading to exposure of collagen with subsequent platelet adherence and aggregation forming the nidus of a thrombus. According to this concept, aspirin, by interfering with the interaction between platelets and collagen, might be expected to reduce the incidence of thrombosis. There is an alternative concept which may perhaps better explain the observed differences in therapy. This argument is based on the idea that it is the generation of thrombin in stagnant blood in the venous valve pockets, and not endothelial damage, which initiates thrombosis (Hume *et al.*, 1970). Stasis plays a primary role in causing venous thrombosis, and it is in the valve pockets of the vein that stasis appears to be maximal. Blood remaining in the leg veins of bed-ridden patients for many minutes would not be cleared of activated blood clotting factors by the liver (Deykin, 1966), thus permitting the formation of trace amounts of thrombin. Such thrombin would induce primary aggregation of platelets directly and also indirectly via the formation of fibrin monomer, despite the presence of aspirin. The apparent failure of aspirin as a prophylactic agent against venous thrombosis thus becomes explicable. Conversely, heparin, even in low doses, would be expected to be highly effective in preventing venous thrombi, if the generation of thrombin were the crucial initiating step in the development of venous thrombi. This has indeed been found to be the case, using a labelled fibrinogen test for detecting venous thrombosis (Kakkar *et al.*, 1971).

On current evidence, therefore, it seems highly unlikely that aspirin represents effective alternative therapy for patients requiring prophylaxis against venous thromboembolism. A similar conclusion may well apply to other drugs which act purely by interfering with the platelet release reaction.

CONCLUSIONS

The weight of evidence indicates that prophylactic anticoagulant therapy properly employed—started before operation and without inordinate delay after admission to hospital—is the most effective and well-proved method of preventing venous thrombosis. The role of dextran is still uncertain. It may well be a useful alternative and does seem to reduce the incidence of thromboembolism in most studies. However, whether dextran is as effective as optimal anticoagulant prophylaxis remains to be determined. Finally, the evidence that platelet-active agents, such as aspirin and dipyridamole, effectively reduce the incidence of pulmonary embolism is unconvincing, and these agents probably should not be used for the prophylaxis of venous thrombosis, except as part of a clinical trial.

TREATMENT

VENOUS THROMBOSIS

In relation to the treatment of established deep vein thrombosis, there are few well-controlled studies. There seems little to be gained by distinguishing between deep and superficial thrombophlebitis in relation to drug treatment, particularly in high-risk patients. While evidence of involvement of the deep veins is a more urgent and serious condition, requiring longer treatment, it is dangerous to accept the converse of this argument, namely that because superficial thrombophlebitis is usually a benign and self-limiting condition, it does not require active treatment. The treatment of choice has been intravenous heparin initially followed by oral anticoagulants for some weeks in the case of deep vein thrombosis. However, while heparin rapidly relieves symptoms, it does not clear the vein of thrombus, nor does it preserve the competency of the venous valves. It is in this area, therefore, that thrombolytic therapy may be of help. In a trial of 30 patients, Kakkar and his colleagues (1969) compared the effects of heparin, streptokinase and ancrod by phlebography and scanning following the injection of labelled fibrinogen. Streptokinase was the most successful form of therapy as judged by the clearance of the occluded vein. Of even greater importance was the observation that, in those patients who were treated with streptokinase within a day or two of the onset of symptoms, the competency of the venous valves was preserved. The prompt induction of a thrombolytic state in deep vein thrombosis will not only relieve symptoms but may prevent subsequent venous insufficiency. Confirmation and extension of these findings may well lead to thrombolytic therapy becoming the treatment of choice for acute venous thrombosis in most patients.

PULMONARY EMBOLISM

Heparin. In patients in whom overt pulmonary embolism has occurred, oral drugs are inadequate to meet this potentially critical situation, because of the time they take to have a significant antithrombotic effect. It has, of course, been known for many years that intravenous heparin is highly effective in the treatment of acute pulmonary embolism. However, recent experimental work has partially explained why this therapy is so effective, and has given some insight into the mechanism of action of heparin in pulmonary embolic disease. Dogs subjected to thromboemboli develop acute airway constriction, due to marked narrowing of the terminal airways; this is not so much bronchospasm as distal airway obstruction. If the animal were given heparin before thrombi were released, airway constriction did not develop following embolisation (Thomas *et al.*, 1964). An important clue to the cause of the airway constriction was provided by examining thrombi before and after embolisation. Stasis thrombi consist of a mesh of fibrin, red cells and scattered platelets. When such thrombi were released to the pulmonary circulation and recovered at autopsy a few minutes later, they had acquired a distinct coating of degranulated platelets (Thomas et al., 1966). However, in animals given heparin no platelet coating developed, and the emboli had the appearance of stasis thrombi. Thus heparin prevented both platelet accretion on an embolus and airway constriction. The link between these two observations is the aggregation of platelets by thrombin with release of their contents. Platelets contain adenine nucleotides, serotonin, histamine, catecholamines and prostaglandins (Holmsen et al., 1969; Smith and Willis, 1971). Several of these substances, once they are released from platelets into the surrounding plasma, can cause constriction of smooth muscle. As blood streams past a partially obstructing thromboembolus, sufficient thrombin is still adsorbed to the clot to cause accretion of platelets on the surface, and release of the platelet contents into an obstructed pulmonary circulation. Thus, with a fresh thromboembolus the problem may not be so much the embolus, but the potent enzyme that is adsorbed to it. Thrombin not only aggregates platelets; it also causes an embolus to propagate via conversion of fibrinogen to fibrin, and it is this secondary thrombosis which completely closes the vessel, as Welch recognised many years ago (Welch, 1899).

These experimental observations help to explain why heparin is so effective in the treatment of acute pulmonary embolism, for it is a potent antithrombin and neutralises almost immediately any thrombin that may be present. Heparin is specific therapy in this context, for it inhibits both propagation and the platelet release reaction. Clinical experience demonstrates that, if rapid treatment with intravenous heparin is instituted, most patients can tolerate even major emboli. This is because heparin has the effect of 'defusing' an embolus, rendering it relatively harmless.

It is interesting to compare the conclusions derived from this experimental work with the much older clinical observations that have been made since heparin was first used in patients in 1935. Swedish workers have, of course, claimed for many years that pulmonary thromboembolism requires treatment with up to 100,000 units of heparin intravenously in the first 24 hours after a major embolus. The ability of heparin to prevent death following pulmonary embolism is attested to by many studies (Jorpes, 1946). When all due allowance is made for the fact that these were mostly uncontrolled trials, and the diagnosis was made by less sophisticated criteria than we would use today, the results are impressive. In the only prospective controlled trial that has been carried out in patients with overt pulmonary embolism, 6 intravenous doses of 10,000 units of heparin were given at 6 hourly intervals, followed by a rapidly acting oral anticoagulant drug (Barritt and Jordan, 1960). In the control group there were 5 deaths and 5 recurrences, whereas in the anticoagulant group there was 1 in-hospital death and no recurrences. The effectiveness of heparin therapy in venous thromboembolism has also been confirmed in more recent studies (Kernohan and Todd, 1966; O'Sullivan et al., 1968).

If heparin is indeed specific therapy, then it follows that a sense of urgency must be brought to the therapeutic management of this disease. A dose of intravenous heparin should be given before time-consuming diagnostic techniques are undertaken, beyond those required at the bedside to make a clinical diagnosis. Heparin should be given in amounts adequate to prevent a platelet-thrombin interaction. Approximately 200 units/kg of heparin were required to prevent platelet accretion on an experimental embolus and it is likely that a similar dose level is required to prevent propagation (Gurewich et al., 1968). If the above reasoning is applied to clinical pulmonary embolism, 10,000–15,000 units should be given intravenously. Furthermore, this regimen should be continued for at least the first 24 hours after the acute episode, giving this dose intravenously every 4 hours to maintain a high blood level. Hence, 60,000 units is a minimum dose of heparin for the first 24 hours. Thereafter, it is reasonable to give lower doses, because less heparin is required to prevent further thrombosis once the acute thrombotic phase has been controlled. Clotting times undoubtedly will be considerably prolonged on this regimen, as would be expected. A daily clotting time may be performed to ensure that the patient is getting enough heparin, but not primarily because of the fear that too much is being given. In the first critical hours, more harm is likely to come from too little heparin than from too much. After the first critical 24–48 hours, sufficient heparin should be given to keep the clotting time prolonged to at least twice the control level, when measured immediately before the next dose is due. However, no controlled trials have been performed to allow a claim that one heparin regimen is superior to the next. A note of caution is warranted in post-menopausal women who have a relatively high incidence of haemorrhagic complications (Jick et al., 1968). In these patients it is prudent to stop heparin as soon as possible, and continue therapy with an oral anticoagulant drug. For most patients, however, heparin and warfarin should overlap for at least 5 days, so that all four clotting factors are depressed to the therapeutic range. Careful avoidance of aspirin and aspirin-containing compounds is essential while a patient is on anticoagulant, and particularly heparin, therapy. The combination of aspirin and heparin dangerously impairs the body's haemostatic defences, and the often inadvertent simultaneous administration of both agents is responsible for many haemorrhagic complications.

Thrombolytic therapy. Two studies recently have reported a comparison between thrombolytic therapy and heparin in the treatment of pulmonary embolism. In Phase 1 of the multicentre co-operative Urokinase Pulmonary Embolism Trial (UPET) study, 160 patients were randomly allocated into either heparin treatment alone or heparin plus 12 hours of urokinase. No significant difference was found in the 2-week mortality rate between the 2 groups of patients (9 per cent in the heparin-treated patients and 7 per cent in the urokinase patients). Similarly, there was no significant difference in the incidence of recurrent pulmonary emboli (19 per cent versus 15 per cent). While there was a statistically significant improvement in the 24 hour pulmonary arteriograms, lung scans and haemodynamic measurements in patients given urokinase, these differences were not reflected in the morbidity and mortality rates. It has been suggested (Hyers *et al.*, 1970) that a proper evaluation of the effect of thrombolytic therapy on mortality from pulmonary embolism requires a trial which includes a large number of patients in shock with massive embolism; possibly a longer period of treatment would also be needed. However, there is little reason to believe that longer treatment with thrombolytic therapy of more severely ill patients is likely to be more successful than heparin in reducing the acute mortality from pulmonary embolism. For example, Miller *et al.* (1971) have recently reported their experience in 23 patients with acute massive pulmonary embolism, treated either with heparin or 72 hours of streptokinase. While haemodynamic and arteriographic findings after treatment showed a significantly greater improvement in the 15 patients given streptokinase, as compared to the 8 patients given heparin, there was in fact no mortality in either group. This study again emphasises the effectiveness of heparin therapy even in patients with massive pulmonary embolism.

The crux of the issue of the role of thrombolytic therapy in pulmonary embolism, as Miller *et al.* (1971) recognise, is that it has yet to be shown that accelerated lysis of emboli produces any therapeutic benefit to the patient. In 1968, Thomas and Gurewich commented that, provided patients survive the initial insult, and provided they are treated with heparin in adequate doses without delay, the prognosis following pulmonary embolism is excellent. They suggested that it was of little consequence whether an embolus was lysed quickly or slowly, and the rapidity of lysis did not usually appear to be a decisive factor in this disease. The data available so far from clinical trials have tended to confirm this viewpoint. It is worth noting that, if the assessment of patients in the UPET study had relied solely on clinical criteria, such as symptoms and signs, routine X-rays, and morbidity and mortality rates, no discernible differences would have emerged between the two groups of patients.

Further experience with thrombolytic drugs in this disease may well delineate a group of patients who would benefit from such treatment—for example, the occasional patient who continues to deteriorate after adequate heparin therapy. However, it is already clear that the contribution of thrombolytic therapy to the treatment of pulmonary embolism is likely to be very limited. Unless some long-term benefit emerges, indicating that lysing an embolus in days instead of weeks is a desirable objective, then heparin is likely to remain the drug of choice for the great majority of patients with acute pulmonary embolism, not least because it is much cheaper and probably safer than thrombolytic therapy.

Ancrod. A coagulant fraction prepared from the venom of the Malayan Pit-Viper, *Ancistrodon rhodostoma* (ancrod) has attracted considerable interest in recent years. This preparation specifically attacks fibrinogen, converting it into a loose fibrin polymer. Ancrod has an action on fibrinogen similar to thrombin, but differs in that it does not split off fibrinopeptide B from the fibrinogen molecule, and does not activate Factor XIII. Ancrod is also dissimilar from thrombin in that it does not attack Factor V and Factor VIII, nor does it cause platelet aggregation. Administration of ancrod intravenously results in a rapid fall in the level of plasma fibrinogen, with the formation of loose fibrin clots. These are quickly removed from the circulation by the fibrinolytic system, with the concomitant formation of fibrin degradation products. Two to three units of ancrod per kg given intravenously over a 4–6 hour period, followed by 2 units per kg every 12 hours, regularly produces and maintains a fibrinogen level of 50 mg per cent or less. Early uncontrolled studies indicated favourable responses to ancrod in some patients with venous thrombosis (Bell *et al.*, 1968; Sharp *et al.*, 1968). In the only controlled trial that has so far been reported, in which ancrod was compared with streptokinase and heparin in the treatment of deep vein thrombosis, ancrod was not significantly superior to heparin (Kakkar *et al.*, 1969). There is some evidence, however, that the incidence of bleeding may be less with ancrod, as compared to heparin.

Only further experience will decide whether the claimed advantages of ancrod (such as standard dosage, simplicity of laboratory control and decreased incidence of bleeding) outweigh the disadvantages (slow induction, cost and occasional development of resistance). While ancrod is undoubtedly a most interesting drug, employing a novel therapeutic approach, it is difficult at present to define a significant role for it in venous thromboembolic disease. It seems unlikely to displace the oral anticoagulants in the field of prophylaxis, it is less effective than thrombolytic drugs in acute venous thrombosis and it acts too slowly to replace heparin in the immediate management of acute pulmonary embolism.

CONCLUSIONS

The vast experience that has accumulated over the years with anticoagulant drugs has shown that, if properly used, the overall mortality rate in patients with clinically diagnosed acute pulmonary embolism is approximately 5 per cent. Such therapy is therefore highly effective for the great majority of patients with venous thromboembolism. Furthermore, it is reasonably safe, relatively inexpensive and its use is firmly based on a wealth of experimental and clinical observations. Anticoagulant therapy therefore remains the basis of our therapeutic approach to venous thromboembolism, and is a standard against which newer methods of therapy must be compared.

There is no reason to believe that the main complication of anticoagulant therapy, namely haemorrhage, is not also a factor with thrombolytic therapy. Indeed, the incidence of haemorrhage in patients given either streptokinase or urokinase appears to be somewhat higher than in patients given anticoagulant therapy. This would be acceptable, if it could be demonstrated that some unequivocal therapeutic benefit resulted from thrombolytic therapy in pulmonary embolism; so far, such evidence has not been forthcoming. However, preliminary experience suggests that thrombolytic therapy may well have a useful role to play in the treatment of acute deep vein thrombosis.

Ancrod has received insufficient controlled trial to decide whether it has a significant therapeutic role in venous thromboembolism. The advantages of ancrod over heparin do not appear to be sufficiently compelling to suggest that it is likely to be a superior therapeutic agent. If the claim that it has a lower incidence of haemorrhage is substantiated, then ancrod may be a useful alternative drug in those patients who are known to be most at risk from haemorrhage when given heparin, for example elderly female patients.

While the future will undoubtedly bring better drugs than are currently available for the control of venous thrombosis and pulmonary embolism, the full and proper use of existing drugs would do much to reduce the toll of this disease.

REFERENCES

BARRITT, D. W. and JORDAN, J. C. (1960) *Lancet*, **1,** 1309.
BELL, W. R. *et al.* (1968) *Lancet*, **1,** 490.
BRISMAN, R. *et al.* (1971) *Ann. Surg.*, **174,** 137.
BRONGE, A. *et al.* (1971) *Acta Chir. Scand.*, **137,** 29.
BYGDEMAN, S. *et al.* (1970) *Lancet*, **2,** 419.
DEYKIN, D. (1966) *J. Clin. Invest.*, **45,** 256.
GUREWICH, V. *et al.* (1968) *Amer. Heart J.*, **76,** 784.
HARRIS, W. H. *et al.* (1967) *J. Bone Jt. Surg.*, **49A,** 81.
HARRIS, W. H. (1971) Personal Communication.
HOLMSEN, H. *et al.* (1969) *Scand. J. Haematol.*, Suppl. 8.
HUME, M. *et al.* (1970) *Venous Thrombosis and Pulmonary Embolism.* Cambridge, Mass.: Harvard University Press.
HYERS, T. M. *et al.* (1970) *Circulation*, **42,** 979.
JICK, H. *et al.* (1968) *New Eng. J. Med.*, **279,** 284.
JORPES, J. E. (1946) *Heparin in the treatment of thrombosis: an account of its chemistry, physiology and application in medicine*, 2nd edition. London: Oxford University Press.
KAKKAR, V. V. *et al.* (1969) *Brit. med. J.* **1,** 806.
KAKKAR, V. V. *et al.* (1971) *Lancet*, **2,** 669.
KAKKAR, V. V. (1972) Personal communication.
KERNOHAN, R. J. and TODD, C. (1966) *Lancet*, **1,** 621.
LAMBIE, J. M. *et al.* (1970) *Brit. med. J.*, **2,** 144.
MILLER, G. A. H. *et al.* (1971) *Brit. med. J.*, **2,** 681.
O'BRIEN, J. R. *et al.* (1971) *Lancet*, **1,** 399.
O'SULLIVAN, E. F. *et al.* (1968) *Med. J. Aust.*, **2,** 153.
SALZMAN, E. W. *et al.* (1971) *New Engl. J. Med.*, **284,** 1287.
SEVITT, S. and GALLAGHER, N. G. (1959) *Lancet*, **2,** 122.
SHARP, A. A. *et al.* (1968) *Lancet*, **1,** 493.
SMITH, J. B. and WILLIS, A. L. (1971) *Nature, New Biology*, **231,** 235.
THOMAS, D. P. *et al.* (1964) *Amer. J. Physiol.*, **206,** 1207.
THOMAS, D. P. *et al.* (1966) *New Engl. J. Med.*, **274,** 953.
THOMAS, D. P. and GUREWICH, V. (1968) *New Engl. J. Med.*, **278,** 338.
Urokinase Pulmonary Embolism Trial (1970) *J. Amer. med. Assoc.*, **214,** 2163.
VANE, J. R. (1971) *Nature, New Biology*, **231,** 232.
WELCH, W. H. (1899) *A System of Medicine*, ed. Allbutt, C. **6,** 228. London: Macmillan.

15 Treatment of Deep Vein Thrombosis with Streptokinase

V. V. Kakkar and P. T. Flute

INTRODUCTION

If the mortality due to pulmonary embolism and morbidity due to the postphlebitic syndrome are to be significantly reduced, there are at least two basic requirements. First, deep vein thrombosis must be diagnosed in all patients and this should be done at an early stage. Second, there must be rapid and complete dissolution of the thrombus at the earliest moment, with preservation of valvular function. There is still a great deal of controversy as to how these treatment aims can be achieved. When conventional anticoagulants are used to treat deep vein thrombosis, they can only reduce the tendency to fresh fibrin formation; the actual removal of the fibrin is left to the spontaneous process of fibrinolysis. While this is sometimes adequate, it is not directly effected by the treatment, and large veins often fail to recanalise or only do so with damage and incompetent valves, in either case leaving permanent disability or the post-phlebitic syndrome. There are, therefore, certain theoretical advantages in using an agent, such as streptokinase, which is known to activate fibrinolysis. The fibrin and fibrinogen degradation products (F.D.P.) which it produces also have a potent anticoagulant effect, especially in the critical early stage.

Trials of streptokinase for arterial disorders have shown that the chances of success are increased if the thrombus is less than 72 hours old, if a continuous infusion is given for several days, and if the dose of streptokinase is sufficient to give such high blood activator levels that there is almost complete removal of circulating plasminogen (Verstraete et al., 1966).

Encouraging results have been reported by the use of streptokinase in the treatment of deep vein thrombosis. With few exceptions (Robertson et al., 1967; 1968; Kakkar et al., 1969a; Mavor, 1970), the majority of previous studies have relied on clinical signs for evaluation of treatment. These have been shown to be misleading, for clinical clearance of symptoms is often complete, despite persisting thrombi within the veins (Kakkar et al., 1969a).

The purpose of this paper is to report the results of treatment in 38 patients with extensive deep vein thrombosis who received streptokinase infusion. Two objective methods were used, as well as careful clinical observation, to study the fate of thrombi. The presence of the thrombus was confirmed in each case by ascending functional phlebography (Kakkar and Flanc, 1968), and this was repeated frequently during treatment. The ^{125}I-fibrinogen test, known to be effective in diagnosing thrombosis (Atkins and Hawkins, 1965; Flanc et al., 1968; Negus et al., 1968), was extended by repeated observations to follow the decline in radioactivity concentrated over the thrombus. Repeated phlebograms have shown that the decline corresponds, for the most part, to the dissolution of thrombi (Kakkar et al., 1968; 1969a, b).

MATERIALS AND METHODS

SELECTION OF PATIENTS

Patients were considered for streptokinase treatment if they had signs and symptoms of deep vein thrombosis which had first appeared in the legs within the preceding 4 days. Because the risk of bleeding would be accentuated at sites of already damaged vessels, no patient was treated within 3 days of operation or when extensive skin flaps were considered unhealed. Similarly, patients with active peptic ulcers and those with a diastolic pressure greater than 100 mm Hg or known to have cerebral vascular haemorrhage or those who had procedures such as lumbar puncture, were exlcuded from this study. All patients were examined by ascending functional phlebography; only when this confirmed the presence of thrombi in the deep veins of the leg was the patient considered suitable for treatment. Occlusion of the tibial and popliteal veins was confirmed by phlebography in every case. Thrombi were also shown in the femoral and iliac veins.

ADMINISTRATION OF STREPTOKINASE

A purified preparation, Kabikinase, kindly supplied by Kabi Pharmaceuticals Limited, was given by continuous intravenous infusion. A loading dose of 500,000 units was given over the first 30 minutes. This was dissolved in 250 ml of 5 per cent glucose and 0·18 per cent saline and given as a slow infusion. The maintenance dose varied in this study; each of the first 8 patients received 100,000 units of streptokinase every hour; subsequently this maintenance dose was increased to 150,000 units hourly. Infusion with streptokinase was continued for a period of 7 days, unless phlebograms showed either complete clearance of thrombus or that there had been no further improvement.

OTHER DRUGS

The first 10 patients in this study received 100 mg of hydrocortisone acetate intravenously 30 minutes before the loading dose. In the remaining patients, 10 mg of chlorpheniramine maleate (Piriton) was used in place of hydrocortisone. This was dissolved in 20 ml of normal saline and was given intravenously before starting the loading dose. At the end of the infusion of streptokinase, intravenous heparin was given for the first 48 hours, and oral anticoagulants, started at the same time, were continued for a minimum period of 4-6 weeks.

ASSESSMENT OF PROGRESS

Clinical. Patients were examined daily, and particular attention was paid to the extent of tenderness, the measured circumference of the limbs at various levels, their temperature, and the appearance of any new symptoms. The vital signs were recorded hourly for 24 hours, then every 4 hours throughout the period of infusion.

Radiographic. The technique of ascending functional phlebography was used; the accuracy of this technique in demonstrating venous thrombi has been described in detail elsewhere (Kakkar and Flanc, 1968; Nicolaides et al., 1971). Briefly, the technique consists of the patient being examined in a horizontal position on a mobile table. Then 30-40 ml of 45 per cent sodium diatriazoate are injected into a vein on the dorsum of the great toe and the contrast medium is diverted into the deep veins by an inflated cuff encircling the ankle. A second cuff is placed in the mid-thigh region and is inflated. The progress of the contrast medium is followed by screening with the aid of an image intensifier and closed circuit television. Once the deep veins are seen to be filled, several films of the calf and thigh regions are exposed in anterio-posterior and lateral views. At this stage, the proximal tourniquet in the mid-thigh region is released. This allows filling of the common iliac veins in each and every patient. In this study, the procedure was repeated at about 48 to 72-hour intervals during treatment and a final phlebogram was performed at the end of therapy.

Isotopic. In 14 patients there was definite evidence of a localised increase in radioactivity at the site of thrombus before treatment. In these patients the thyroid gland was first blocked by sodium iodide (100 mg) given intravenously half an hour prior to the injection of ^{125}I-labelled fibrinogen (100 μci). Radioactive counting was performed along the leg after 1 hour and again after 6–12 hours and then daily during the streptokinase infusion. The details of the counting procedure were those previously described (Flanc et al., 1968). Repeated counts of radioactivity over the site of thrombus and over areas where there were no thrombi allowed a quantitative assessment of the fate of the thrombus (Kakkar et al., 1968; 1969a). The decrease in the percentage difference of radioactivity over these two sites indicated the rate of thrombus dissolution; this was confirmed by repeated phlebography.

Laboratory studies. In 10 patients, detailed laboratory investigations were undertaken to see if the dose of streptokinase given had produced certain definite effects. Samples of venous blood were collected in one-tenth volume of 3·8 per cent trisodium citrate before the start of treatment, half an hour after the loading dose of streptokinase, and at daily intervals thereafter. These were used for estimation of streptokinase inhibitors (Flute, 1964a) before starting treatment, and for measurement of fibrinogen, plasminogen, dilute blood clot lysis time, and activity of the euglobulin fraction of plasma on unheated bovine fibrin plates (Flute, 1964b). Fibrin and fibrinogen degradation products (F.D.P.) were measured by the tanned red cell haemagglutination inhibition technique (Merskey et al., 1966). Prothrombin time, partial thromboplastin time and thrombin clotting time were measured by standard techniques (Hardisty and Ingram, 1965). Platelet function was studied as described by Hutton and O'Shea (1968).

RESULTS

CLINICAL RESULTS

Of 38 patients studied, 30 successfully completed the treatment. In 8 patients treatment had to be abandoned because of various reasons. Three patients developed anaphylactic reactions after not more than 10,000 units of streptokinase had been injected. These patients became distressed, with dyspnoea, cyanosis, bronchospasm, tachycardia and fall in blood pressure. The symptoms subsided rapidly on discontinuing the infusion and repeating the dose of hydrocortisone. In none of these patients was there a history of allergic tendencies and in none was there any evidence of recent streptococcal infection. In these 3 patients, inhibitors of streptokinase, which included antibodies to streptokinase, were in the middle range. In another 4 patients severe bleeding prevented an adequate course of treatment being given. In the eighth patient, repeated episodes of hypotension were the reason for discontinuing the treatment on the fifth day.

Clinical signs rapidly disappeared in 26 patients and only 4 of the

30 had any residual symptoms at the end of the treatment. Tenderness disappeared rapidly, often within 12–24 hours but oedema often persisted for some days.

PHLEBOGRAPHIC RESULTS

Of the 26 patients judged to show a successful clinical result, 12 showed complete clearance of all thrombi after treatment for periods varying between 9 hours and 7 days. Symptoms of thrombosis had been present for less than 72 hours before treatment in each of these cases. The remaining 14 patients showed substantial but incomplete thrombolysis, even after 7 days of infusion. Four patients with residual clinical signs still retained their original extensive thrombi.

RADIOACTIVE FIBRINOGEN RESULTS

Fourteen patients had increased uptake of radioactive fibrinogen at the site of the thrombus. The original difference between this and the activity at an adjacent site was taken as 100 per cent. The percentage decline of this difference (thrombus radioactivity) was assumed to represent the degree of disolution of thrombus and this was confirmed by phlebography.

The counts fell to less than 50 per cent within 36 hours in 12 patients treated with streptokinase; in 2 patients who showed no improvement on phlebographic examination, the counts were still greater than 50 per cent after 5 days of treatment.

LABORATORY STUDY RESULTS

The first 10 patients in this study had detailed laboratory investigations. Significant changes in haemoglobulin and P.C.V. were only found in 3 patients with abnormal bleeding. All patients showed considerable fibrinolytic activity of the euglobulin fraction tested on bovine fibrin plates. In the early stages, dilute clot lysis times of less than 10 minutes, were regularly observed, but later lysis times were longer than 7 hours, despite the increased activity in the euglobulin fraction.

Results for plasminogen, fibrinogen and F.D.P. are shown in Table 15.1 and Figure 15.1.

Plasminogen was rapidly depleted, fibrinogen fell, and F.D.P. appeared in very large amounts. F.D.P. had returned to almost normal levels within 48 hours. Thrombin clotting time results ran in parallel with F.D.P. estimations. With a normal control of 10–15 seconds, the time was considerably prolonged for the first 36–48 hours but after this seldom exceeded the control by more than a

TABLE 15.1
LABORATORY RESULTS

Day	No. of samples tested	Fibrinogen (mg per 100 ml)		Fibrinogen degradation products (μg per ml)		Plasminogen (casein units per ml)	
		Mean	Range	Mean	Range	Mean	Range
Before infusion	9	486	305–610	43	9–115	3.5	0.8–5.6
After infusion	5	269	125–405	1604	768–3000	0.6	0–1.4
1	9	208	120–280	769	48–3000	0.4	0–0.9
2	6	197	160–240	96	12–384	Nil	–
3	7	176	125–200	41	12–102	0.5	0–1.1
4	6	138	70–185	73	32–104	0.5	0–1.4
5	3	138	110–165	64	29–104	0.4	0–1.2
6	2	148	135–170	33	14–52	Nil	–
7	1	215	–	24	–	Nil	–

few seconds. Inhibitor levels before treatment varied between 5–60 units of streptokinase per ml of plasma, with a mean of 20 units per ml.

For the first 36 hours platelet adhesion to plasma and aggregation in response to adenosine diphosphate (A.D.P.) and collagen was impaired in the majority of patients investigated.

SIDE EFFECTS

The most frequent side-effect was pyrexia, which occurred in 18 patients who received an infusion lasting longer than 12 hours. The rise in temperature varied from 2°–5.6°F in most cases, was associated with chills and was usually evident about 14–24 hours after infusion began and reached a peak after a further 24–36 hours. Previous administration of hydrocortisone or antihistamines did not seem to alter the frequency of pyrexia. Three patients had allergic reactions which have already been described.

Bleeding was a complication in 10 patients. Minor bleeding occurred in 4 patients, either in the form of subcutaneous haematoma or minor oozing from a groin incision and from a tracheostomy wound. In 6 patients the bleeding was severe enough to require neutralisation of circulating activator with tranexamic acid (Cyklokapron) and fresh blood transfusion.

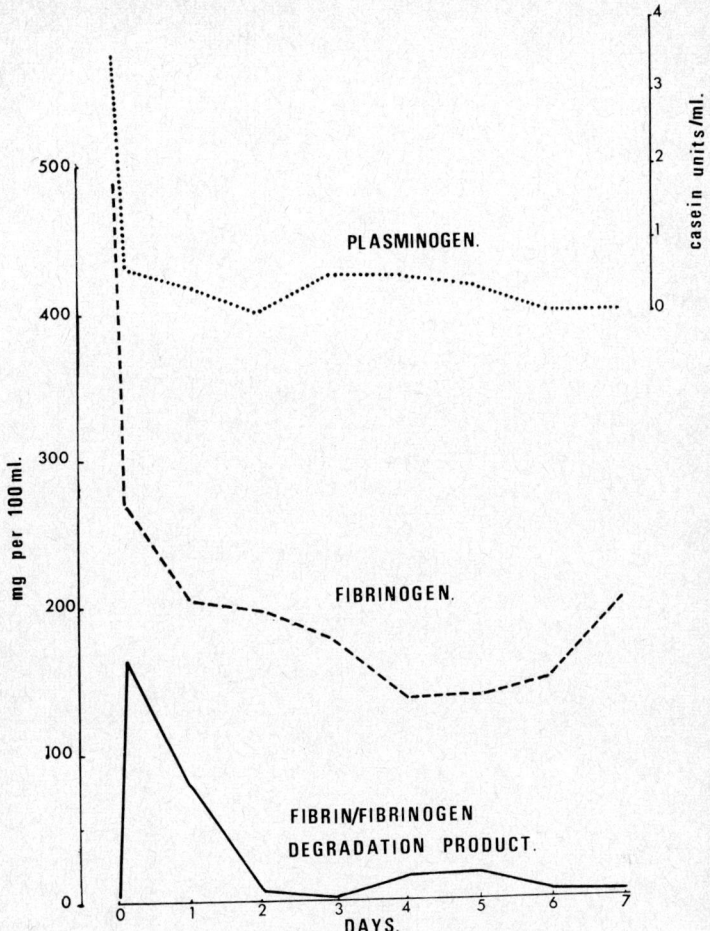

Fig. 15.1. Average laboratory results during streptokinase therapy.

DISCUSSION

There is still a great deal of argument as to which is the best form of medical treatment for patients with extensive deep vein thrombosis. This is largely due to the lack of well-controlled studies where the effectiveness of different treatments has been measured accurately. There have indeed been very few reported studies of treatment in homogeneous groups of patients, where the effect of treatment has been assessed by such objective methods as the radioactive fibrinogen test and phlebography. In one study the course of treatment was compared in three homogeneous groups of patients who were allocated at random to one of three treatment schedules (Kakkar et al., 1969b). One group was given the conventional treatment for this condition, consisting of intravenous heparin administered for a period of 7 days; the second group was treated with the plasminogen activator, streptokinase (Kabikinase) which is known to have a thrombolytic effect (Verstraete et al., 1966; Browse, 1968; Kakkar et al., 1969). The third group was treated with ancrod which has a specific coagulant action on fibrinogen (Bell et al., 1968). The results of treatment were assessed in each group by clinical examination, the radioactive fibrinogen test and phlebography. The results showed that there was little to choose between heparin and ancrod so far as their anticoagulant potential was concerned, except that the risk of haemorrhage appeared to be greater when ancrod was used. Streptokinase was undoubtedly the most effective drug used for inducing a thrombolytic state and, indeed, for lysing the clot. Nevertheless, there are certain disadvantages of streptokinase and it is not always successful. It is highly antigenic in man; as a result of previous streptococcal infection, most individuals tend to have a variable level of circulating streptokinase antibodies. It was considered to be essential to determine this level because sufficient streptokinase should be given not only to neutralise these antibodies, but also to be available in excess for activation of plasminogen. Unless this is taken into consideration, the results of streptokinase therapy will be disappointing (Fletcher et al., 1959). In most people, 500,000 units of streptokinase, given in 30 minutes will neutralise their circulating antibodies and also provide the necessary excess to convert rapidly all the circulating plasminogen to plasmin. If the streptokinase infusion is then continued, giving 100,000 units or more per hour, the only plasminogen available will be that which is freshly synthesised, and this is really insufficient to allow other than minor digestion of plasma proteins. It is our common practice for the loading dose of 500,000 units of streptokinase to be given in 30 minutes, followed by a maintenance dose of 100,000–150,000 units every hour. The dose is dissolved in normal saline and given as a slow infusion.

Injection of streptokinase directly into a thrombus offers the best chance of successful thrombolysis. Nevertheless, systemic administration of large dose usually has been adopted because of the widespread nature of the thrombotic process. Rapid lysis may be obtained in some thrombi, but administration may have to be continued for up to 6 days; even this is not uniformly effective (Kakkar et al., 1968; 1969). Factors known to affect the outcome are the extent and age of the thrombus. Since the activator must reach the surface of the thrombus to produce the desired effect, thrombolysis is achieved more readily in a vessel which is not completely occluded. However, clearance is obtained in many veins which have been completely occluded by thrombus (Robertson et al., 1968, 1969; Kakkar et al., 1969; Madar et al., 1970). The age of the thrombus seems to be more important than its extent; the best results are obtained when the thrombi have been present for less than 36 hours before treatment is commenced.

Good results can, however, be obtained up to something like 72 hours after initiation of thrombosis—indeed, worthwhile results may occasionally be obtained after this where the new part of the thrombus is lysed, but the older and organised part remains. The worst results occur when there is continuing stimulus to fibrin formation, such as inflammation localised around the veins, for example in the pelvis (Kakkar et al., 1969b; 1970).

There are certain disadvantages in using streptokinase; immediate allergic reaction and pyrexia are not uncommon and sometimes have been troublesome. Prophylactic hydrocortisone administration may not control these effectively. Because of the risk of haemorrhage, close laboratory supervision is required to give forewarning of a likely bleeding episode. This would perhaps be most obvious when the presence of excessive products of fibrinogen lysis have caused an unusual prolongation of thrombin clotting time.

A further disadvantage of streptokinase is its ability to form neutralising antibodies in high titre which, for a time at least, would preclude a second course of treatment in the same patient (Flute, 1964b).

Specific contraindications to streptokinase therapy are the same as those for any anticoagulant regime. However, there are situations where the possibility of bleeding must be weighed carefully against the risk of fatal pulmonary embolism. Drugs such as streptokinase should be used with caution in patients within 72 hours of major surgical operations, or even longer if there are extensive raw areas of granulation tissue which can act as the locus for active haemorrhage.

Since the available forms of treatment are not always safe nor invariably effective, it is wise to restrict their use to selected patients. The natural history of deep vein thrombosis clearly indicates that patients with spreading thrombosis, with involvement of the popliteal or even more proximal veins, require active treatment for at least two reasons: first, there is a significant risk of pulmonary embolism in such cases (Kakkar et al., 1969b). Secondly, with more extensive involvement of the deep veins, there is an increasing risk of the late sequelae of the postphlebitic syndrome.

The value of streptokinase in preventing the postphlebitic syndrome has yet to be determined. Streptokinase, which actively lyses the thrombus, is the most effective agent available at present for preserving valvular function. In a recent study (Kakkar et al., 1969c), patients with deep vein thrombosis who had been treated during the acute phase with different therapies, were further investigated in an attempt to answer the following questions:

1. What form of initial treatment was most successful in achieving eventual normal valvular function?
2. What are the critical factors involved in preserving the function of venous valves?

Ascending functional cinephlebography, specially devised to observe valvular function, was used in 22 patients restudied after intervals of up to 12 months after initial treatment with heparin, streptokinase or ancrod (Table 15.2).

TABLE 15.2

LATE RESULTS

Valvular Function up to 12 Months after Initial Treatment

Initial treatment	Number of patients	Valvular function		
		Normal	Poor	Absent
Heparin	8	1	1	6
Streptokinase	7	4	1	2
Ancrod	7	0	1	6
All	22	5	3	14

Early diagnosis was found to be of paramount importance; at this stage, organisation of thrombus had not taken place and complete lysis was possible. To be as certain as possible of preserving valvular function the diagnosis must be made within 36-48 hours of the onset of thrombosis, and the thrombus dissolved rapidly. When heparin or ancrod were used, the initial clearance of veins was slower and less complete, and subsequent valvular function less satisfactory. The number of patients investigated in this study was small and therefore no definite conclusions could be drawn. The findings do, however, give a hint of the possible benefits of using streptokinase. Work is now in progress where a large number of patients treated with streptokinase are being followed up for longer periods to see if the use of this drug will prevent the late sequelae.

REFERENCES

ATKINS, P. and HAWKINS, L. A. (1965) *Lancet*, **2**, 1217.
BELL, W. R. *et al.* (1968) *Lancet*, **1**, 490.
BROWSE, N. L. and NEGUS, D. (1970) *Brit. med. J.*, **1**, 45.
FLANC, C. *et al.* (1968) *Brit. J. Surg.*, **55**, 742.
FLETCHER, A. P. *et al.* (1965) *J. Lab. Clin. Med.*, **65**, 713.
FLUTE, P. T. (1964a) *Brit. med. Bull.*, **20**, 195.
FLUTE, P. T. (1964b) *Ann. Royal Coll. Surg. Engl.*, **36**, 225.
HARDISTY, R. M. and INGRAM, G. I. C. (1965) *Bleeding Disorders*. Oxford: Blackwell.
HUTTON, R. A. and O'SHEA, M. J. (1968) *J. Clin. Path.*, **21**, 406.
KAKKAR, V. V. and FLANC, C. (1968) *Brit. J. Surg.*, **55**, 384.
KAKKAR, V. V. *et al.* (1969a) *Brit. med. J.*, **56**, 178.
KAKKAR, V. V. *et al.* (1969b) *Brit. med. J.*, **1**, 806.
KAKKAR, V. V. *et al.* (1969c) *Brit. med. J.*, **1**, 810.
MADAR, G. *et al.* (1970) *J. Suisse Med.*, **100**, 1337.
MERSKEY, C. *et al.* (1966) *Blood*, **28**, 1.
NEGUS, D. *et al.* (1968) *Brit. J. Surg.*, **55**, 835.
NICOLAIDES, A. N. *et al.* (1970) *Brit. J. Surg.*, **57**, 860.
ROBERTSON, B. R. *et al.* (1968) *Acta Chir. Scand.*, **134**, 203.
VERSTRAETE, M. *et al.* (1966) *Brit. med. J.*, **1**, 454.

16 Streptokinase and Pulmonary Embolism

G. C. Sutton, G. A. H. Miller, I. H. Kerr,
R. V. Gibson and M. Honey

INTRODUCTION

The natural history of pulmonary embolism is variable, and the factors responsible for individual variation poorly understood. Severity of embolism (i.e. degree of obstruction to the pulmonary vascular bed), duration of embolism, and the presence of pre-existing cardio-respiratory disease may be some of these factors. Some patients who have 'massive' pulmonary embolism die shortly after the event (Gorham, 1961), while others with equally 'massive' embolism survive to lyse their emboli spontaneously (Sautter et al., 1964; Fred et al., 1966; Dalen et al., 1969). Another group of patients with massive pulmonary embolism may survive the initial episode, but die within days or weeks and yet others may survive, fail to lyse their emboli and are left with chronic thrombo embolic pulmonary hypertension. Patients who have 'minor' pulmonary embolism usually recover spontaneously, but occasionally develop important pulmonary complications, or following repetitive small pulmonary emboli develop chronic thrombo embolic pulmonary hypertension. Co-existing additional cardio-pulmonary disease may result in a poorer prognosis for pulmonary embolism than patients who have previously normal cardio-respiratory systems (Murphy and Bullock, 1967) and a slower rate of resolution (Hirsh et al., 1968).

There exist ever-increasing reports of rapid lysis of pulmonary embolism using the fibrinolytic agents streptokinase (Hirsh et al., 1968; Miller et al., 1969) and urokinase (Dickie et al., 1967; Sautter et al., 1967; Sasahara et al., 1967; Tow et al., 1967; Genton and Wolf, 1968; Urokinase Pulmonary Embolism Trial, 1970).

This study was concerned with a group of patients, all of whom had massive pulmonary embolism defined by pulmonary arteriography, all of whom were seen between 2–48 hours following the acute episode, and none of whom had pre-existing cardio-respiratory disease. The objective of the study was to compare the effects of treatment by streptokinase or heparin over a 72-hour period.

TECHNIQUE OF TREATMENT

Following clinical evaluation (Sutton et al., 1969), which included a plain chest X-ray (Kerr et al., 1971) and standard 12-lead electrocardiogram, the patient was transferred to the cardiac catheterisation laboratory where right heart catheterisation was performed under local anaesthesia introducing an angiographic catheter into the right medial cubital vein. Pressures were recorded in the right atrium, right ventricle, and pulmonary artery together with the brachial artery pressure obtained by an indwelling polyethylene cannula. All pressures were referred to the mid-chest level. Cardiac output was measured using the Fick principle, the oxygen consumption in expired air being determined by the micro-Scholander technique (Scholander, 1947). Oxygen saturation in pulmonary and brachial artery samples was measured by reflection oximetry (Zijlstra and Mook, 1962). A single-plane, antero-posterior, pulmonary arteriogram was then performed using 0·5–1 ml/kg body weight of contrast medium injected by a pressure injector.

During the course of treatment (see below), the patient was observed in an intensive care unit with the pulmonary artery catheter used for infusion of heparin or streptokinase direct into the main pulmonary artery. Following a 72-hour period, the patient returned to the catheterisation laboratory for repeat haemodynamic measurements and pulmonary arteriography.

DETAILS OF TREATMENT

The dosage of streptokinase used was 600,000 units in the first half-hour followed by 100,000 units/hour for a total of 72 hours. Estimation of the titrated initial dose (Nilsson and Olow, 1962) indicated that this initial dosage was adequate in all patients. Serial measurements of haemoglobin, prothrombin time, euglobulin lysis time and whole-blood clotting time (Lee and White) were made during treatment. Hydrocortisone 100 mg/6 hourly intravenously was given to prevent the development of febrile reactions.

Heparin was given in a dose adjusted to achieve a clotting time of 20–30 minutes, the dose required varying from 48,000–60,000 units/24 hours.

CHOICE OF TREATMENT

Initially, patients were treated with streptokinase and later with heparin. Although the choice of treatment was never dictated by the clinical condition of the patient, the last 15 patients were allocated randomly to treatment by heparin or streptokinase, the clinician in charge of the patient being ignorant of which drug the patient was receiving.

PATIENTS TREATED

Thirty patients (11 male, 19 female) aged 14–69 years were treated with either heparin (12 patients) or streptokinase (18 patients). There were no important distinctions between the two groups in such pre-treatment clinical factors as a history of circulatory arrest or syncope, the incidence of previous premonitory minor pulmonary emboli, the duration of massive embolism, and the probable age of the venous thrombus. The patients were in approximately equal age groups.

PRE-TREATMENT HAEMODYNAMIC AND ARTERIOGRAPHIC ASSESSMENT

The haemodynamic findings in patients before treatment with either heparin or streptokinase were closely similar in the two groups (Table 16.1).

TABLE 16.1
PRE-TREATMENT HAEMODYNAMIC FINDINGS

There were no significant differences with respect to pulmonary artery systolic pressure, total pulmonary resistance, arterio-venous oxygen (A-V O_2) difference, right ventricular end-diastolic (RVED) pressure, arterial oxygen saturation or cardiac index. (SK = streptokinase—18 patients treated; 12 heparin patients treated). Mean values only shown.

	SK (18)	Heparin (12)
Pulmonary Systolic pressure (mm Hg)	43·7	41·9
Total Pulmonary resistance (units × sq. M)	18·3	16·4
A—VO_2 difference (ml/100^{2}ml)	7·8	7·8
R.V.E.D. (mm Hg)	12·4	12·3
Arterial Saturation (%)	85·6	82·6
Cardiac Index	1·9	1·9

These findings reflect the usual haemodynamic disturbance of acute massive pulmonary embolism in that there was moderate pulmonary hypertension, a wide arterio-venous oxygen difference with a low cardiac output and elevated total pulmonary resistance (Miller and Sutton, 1970; Sutton, 1970). There was right ventricular 'failure', (as judged by a high right ventricular end-diastolic pressure). Arterial oxygen desaturation was a usual finding.

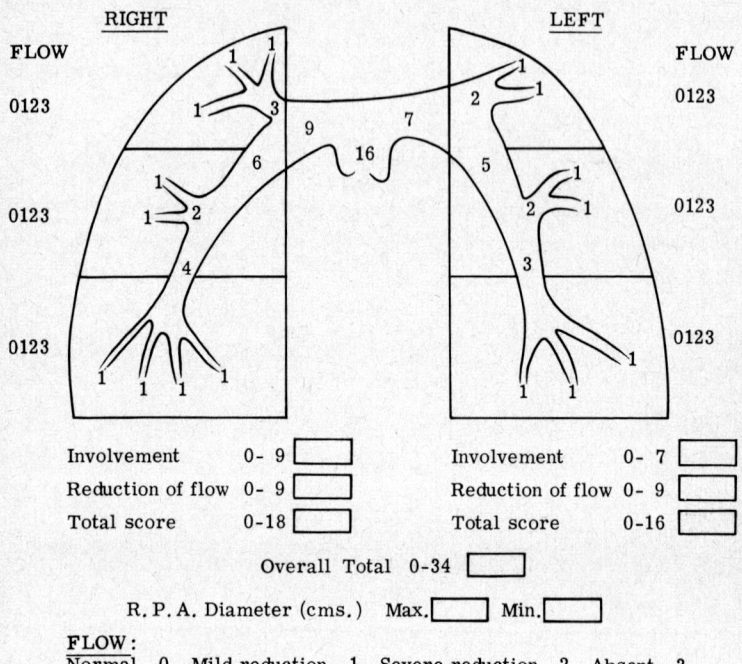

FIG. 16.1. Method of scoring pulmonary arteriogram (see text)

In an attempt to assess arteriographic appearances objectively, all pulmonary arteriograms were scored by a radiologist taking into account both embolic involvement and pulmonary artery 'flow' (Fig. 16.1). The presence of a filling defect proximal to segmental branches of the pulmonary arteries scored a value equal to the number of segmental branches arising distally. Thus a maximum of 16 points was possible for complete involvement of the major pulmonary arteries. The lungs were divided into 6 zones, and flow assessed as absent (3 points), severely reduced (2 points), mildly reduced (1 point) or normal (0), in each zone. A maximum of 18 points for flow reduction was possible. Each arteriogram was therefore scored out of a maximum possible 34 points combining involvement and flow reduction.

There were no significant differences in the pre-treatment mean arteriographic indices of severity in the two treatment groups.

RESULTS

CLINICAL

There was clinical improvement during the 72-hour period of treatment in 25 of the 30 patients. This improvement was particularly striking in the reduction in respiratory rate, and the regression of the physical signs of low cardiac output and right ventricular failure. Such improvement was observed to be more rapid in patients receiving streptokinase than in those receiving heparin.

Five patients deteriorated clinically during treatment: four of these were on heparin, and one on streptokinase. Treatment in these 5 patients had been randomly allocated. The patient receiving streptokinase and two of the four on heparin had successful pulmonary embolectomy with cardio-pulmonary bypass, while the two other patients on heparin were changed to streptokinase therapy, one of whom later had pulmonary emblectomy.

HAEMODYNAMIC

The pre- and post-treatment results for the group as a whole and for the patients randomly allocated to treatment with respect to pulmonary artery systolic pressure and total pulmonary resistance are shown in Figs. 16.2 and 16.3.

It is important to appreciate that these results do not take into account those patients (see above) who did not complete the course of treatment because of clinical deterioration. These results, therefore, are the most favourable possible for either treatment group, and as four patients with heparin and only one with streptokinase were excluded, the results relatively favour the heparin group.

PULMONARY ARTERY SYSTOLIC PRESSURE (FIGURE 16.2)

In the group as a whole, patients treated with streptokinase had a highly significant fall in pulmonary artery systolic pressure (43.7 ± 9.7 mm Hg before treatment, 29.5 ± 7.9 mm Hg following treatment; $p < 0.001$). There was a lesser fall in pulmonary artery systolic pressure in patients treated with heparin (41.9 ± 5.0 mm Hg before treatment, 37.1 ± 8.0 mm Hg after treatment; $p < 0.05$).

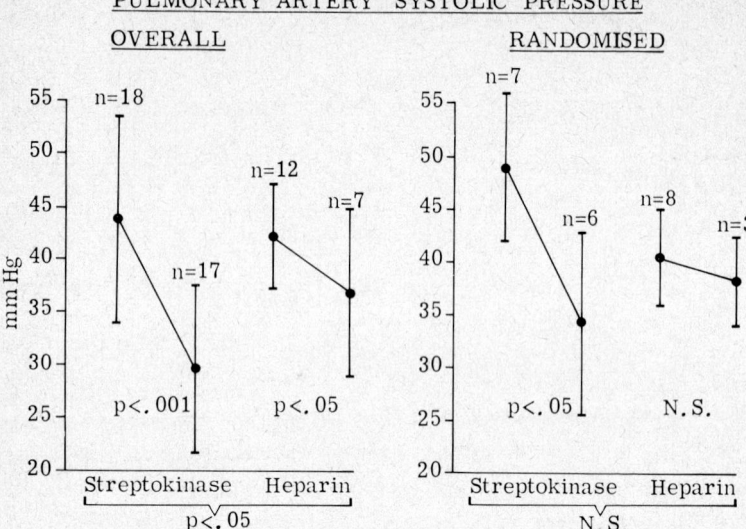

Fig. 16.2. Pulmonary artery systolic pressure: Comparative results (mean ± 1 S.D. shown) for patients treated with streptokinase and heparin. Results for the overall group shown on left, and for randomised patients on right. n = number of patients in whom these measurements could be made before (left) and after (right) treatment. Significant changes are shown. (N.S. = not significant.)

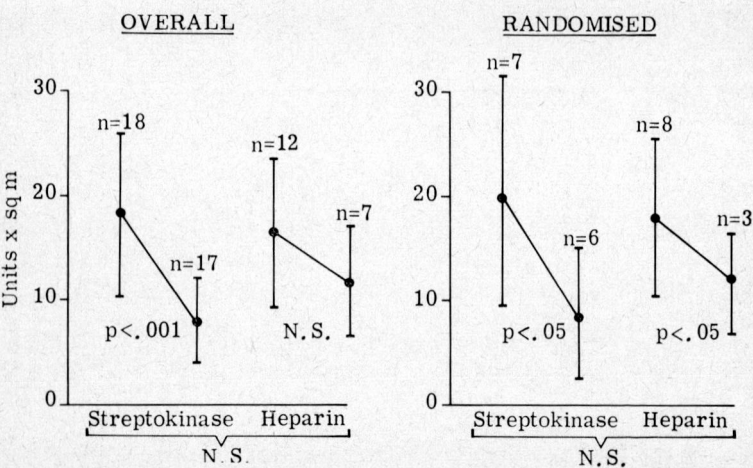

Fig. 16.3. Total pulmonary resistance. Key as for Figure 16.2.

In those patients randomly allocated to treatment, there was a fall in those treated with streptokinase (49.1 ± 7.2 mm Hg before treatment and 34.2 ± 8.6 mm Hg after treatment; $p < 0.05$), but no significant change in those treated with heparin (40.4 ± 4.4 mm Hg before treatment and 38.3 ± 4.1 mm Hg after treatment).

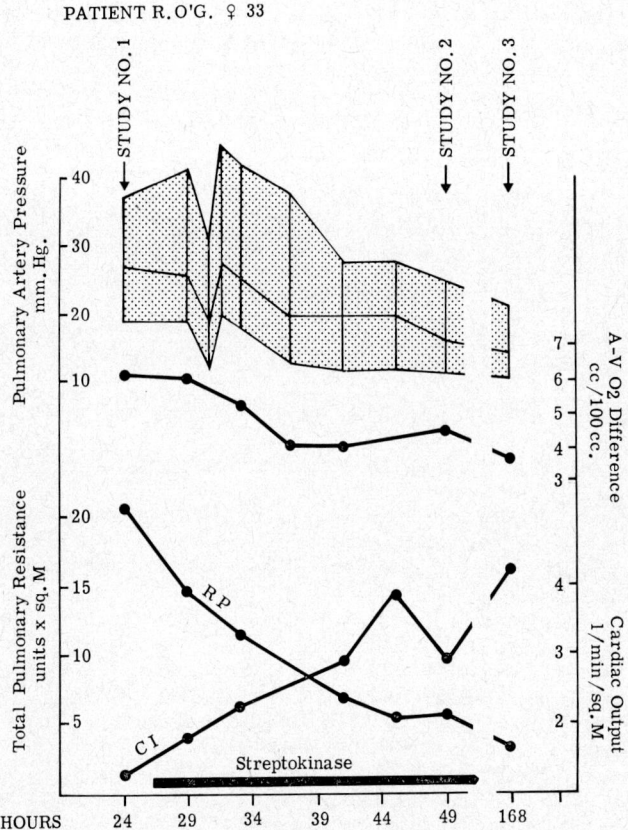

FIG. 16.4. Haemodynamic measurements in a patient treated with streptokinase with treatment starting 26 hours after massive embolism. The haemodynamic findings are within normal limits some 15 hours later. (RP = total pulmonary resistance; C.I. = cardiac index).

TOTAL PULMONARY RESISTANCE (FIGURE 16.3)

In the group as a whole, there was a highly significant fall in total pulmonary resistance in patients treated with streptokinase (18.3 ± 7.7 units $\times$ SqM before treatment and 8.2 ± 4.1 units $\times$ SqM after treatment; $p < 0.001$), while the fall did not achieve significance in those treated with heparin (16.4 ± 6.9 units $\times$ SqM before treatment and 11.9 ± 5.3 units $\times$ SqM after treatment).

In the randomly allocated patients, there was some fall in both treatment groups: (In the streptokinase group, 20.1 ± 11.6 units $\times$ SqM before treatment and 8.8 ± 6.4 units $\times$ SqM after treatment; $p < 0.05$. In the heparin group, 18.1 ± 7.7 units $\times$ SqM before treatment and 11.7 ± 4.5 units $\times$ SqM after treatment; $p < 0.05$).

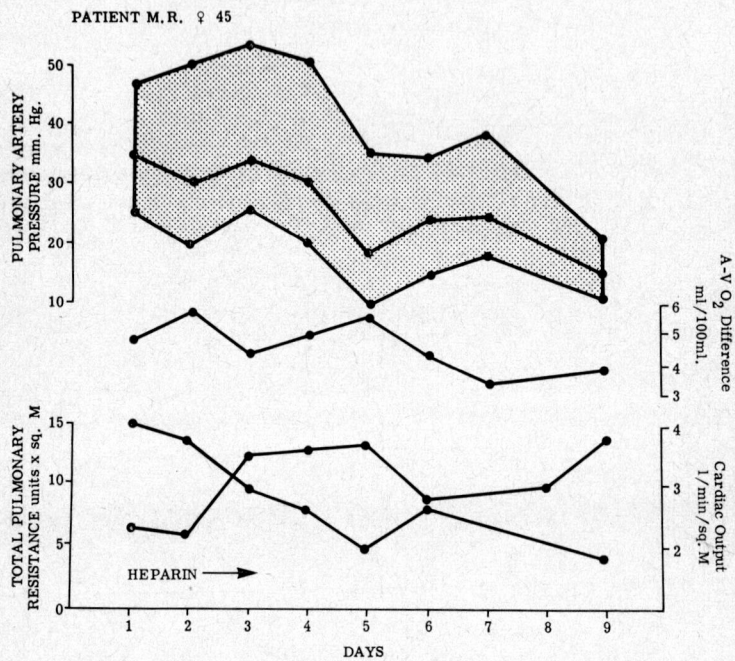

FIG. 16.5. Haemodynamic measurements in a patient treated with heparin. Treatment started 24 hours after massive embolism, with haemodynamic findings becoming normal after 4 days of treatment.

A typical, but not invariable response to treatment with streptokinase is shown in Fig. 16.4. This shows that the pulmonary artery pressure, total pulmonary resistance and arterio-venous oxygen difference have fallen to within normal levels some 15 hours after initiating treatment while the cardiac index has risen. By contrast, although also achieving a normal end-result after 9 days, the improvement has been much slower in a patient treated with heparin (Fig. 16.5).

ANGIOGRAPHIC (FIGURE 16.6)

In the group as a whole, there was a highly significant angiographic improvement in the patients treated with streptokinase after 72 hours (24.3 ± 2.7 units before treatment, 10.2 ± 7.2 units after treatment; $p < 0.001$). There was no significant change in those treated with heparin (24.1 ± 2.8 units and 20.1 ± 5.3 units).

In the randomised patients, the improvement was again significant with streptokinase (24.9 ± 1.5 before treatment and 14.7 ± 6.3 units after treatment; $p < 0.01$), while it was not significant with heparin

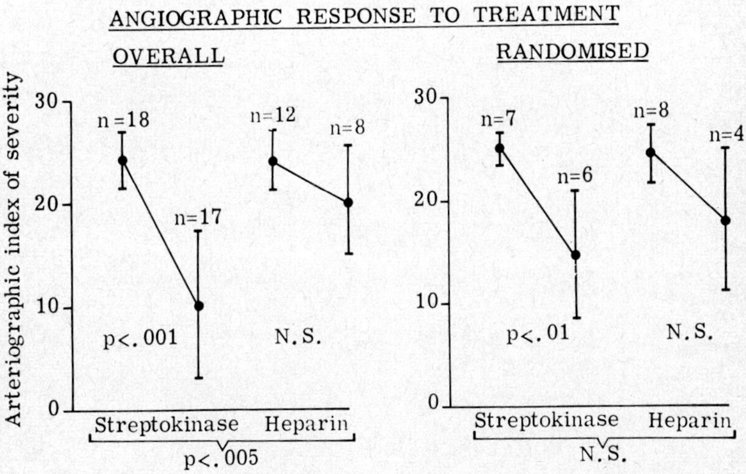

FIG. 16.6. Angiographic response to treatment. Comparative results (mean ± 1 S.D. shown) for streptokinase and heparin using arteriographic index of severity. In the overall results, there is a highly significant improvement with streptokinase, but not with heparin. There is a significant end-point difference between streptokinase and heparin. In the randomised patients, there is significant improvement in streptokinase treated patients, but not in those with heparin.

(24.4 ± 2.9 before treatment and 18.0 ± 6.9 units after treatment). Whereas there was a significant ($p < 0.005$) difference in the angiographic end-result between the groups treated with streptokinase and heparin in the overall series, the end-result had not reached significance in the randomised patients.

Considerable angiographic improvement following 72 hours of treatment with streptokinase is shown in Fig. 16.7, and although not invariable, this illustrated the usual response to streptokinase. By contrast, failure to produce angiographic resolution was the usual experience in patients treated with heparin (Fig. 16.8), although rarely a better result was achieved.

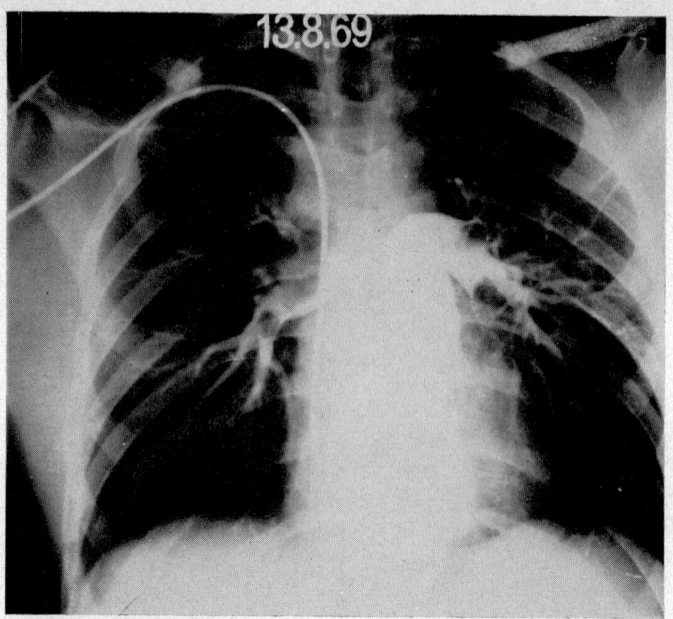
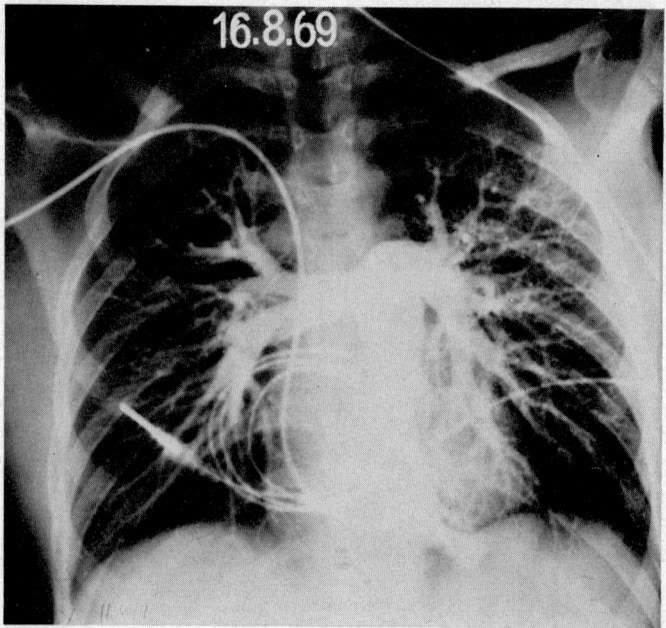

FIG. 16.7. Pulmonary arteriograms taken before (upper) and after (lower) 72 hours treatment with streptokinase showing marked improvement. Pre-treatment arteriographic severity was 27 points, and post-treatment 4 points.

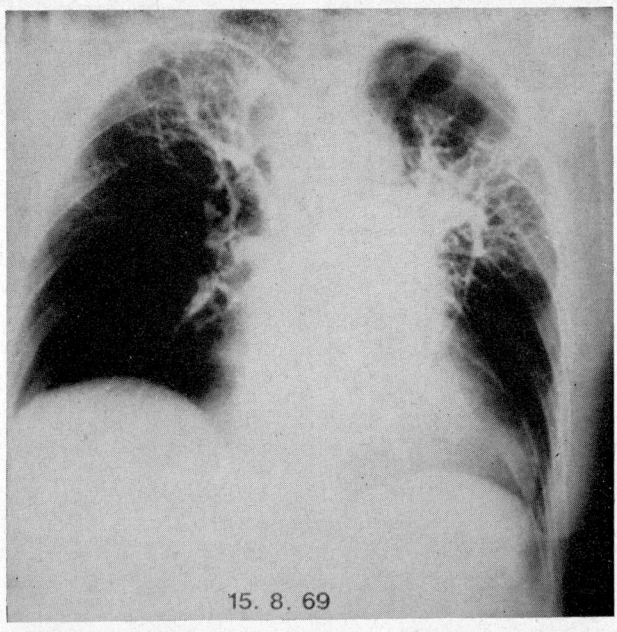
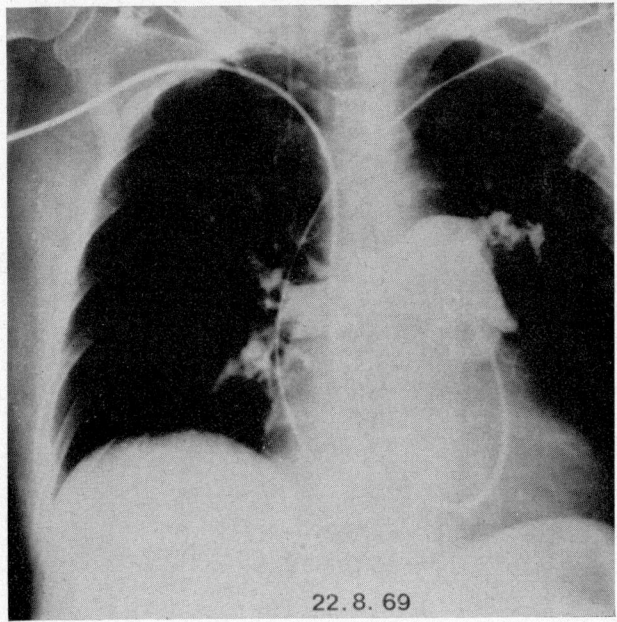

Fig. 16.8. Pulmonary arteriograms taken before (upper) and after (lower) 7 days treatment with heparin. No improvement is seen. Pretreatment score 28 points, post-treatment score 27 points.

COMPLICATIONS AND SIDE-EFFECTS

Bleeding from cut-down or operation sites occurred in 9 patients (50 per cent) receiving streptokinase and 2 patients (16 per cent) receiving heparin. Slight bleeding from other sites occurred in two streptokinase-treated patients, and one heparin-treated patient. There was severe gastro-intestinal bleeding in one heparin-treated patient. Transfusion was necessary in three streptokinase-treated patients and two heparin-treated patients. Streptokinase treatment had to be stopped in one patient because of bleeding. A pyrexia of 38–39°C occurred in four patients receiving streptokinase, and in one patient receiving heparin.

DISCUSSION

This study permits limited conclusions about the relative effects of streptokinase and heparin during a 72-hour treatment period in patients surviving the initial two hours following massive pulmonary embolism. In such patients in whom additional cardio-respiratory disease was not present, there was significantly greater angiographic resolution after 72 hours treatment by streptokinase than by heparin.

The haemodynamic response to treatment by these drugs over a 72-hour period was not markedly different. In general, pulmonary artery pressure fell in patients treated with both streptokinase and heparin, usually achieving normal levels after streptokinase, but remaining elevated in patients treated with heparin. As cardiac output rose in both treatment groups, total pulmonary resistance fell irrespective of treatment choice. Similarly, right ventricular end-diastolic pressure fell, and arterial oxygen saturation rose in the 72-hour treatment period both with streptokinase and heparin. These measured haemodynamic parameters mirror the improved clinical condition of the patient over this same period. In general, however, the response in patients treated with streptokinase has been more rapid than in those treated with heparin, although the end-result after one week may be the same.

An important aspect of these 30 patients is that there was no mortality in either treatment group. This fact emphasises that most of the mortality from massive pulmonary embolism occurs immediately or shortly after the event, while the patients reported here had all survived this critical period before treatment was started. Nevertheless, there were 5 patients (16 per cent) whose condition deteriorated while receiving treatment, four of these on heparin and one on streptokinase. The reasons for this deterioration are not clear but in the absence of evidence for recurrence of pulmonary embolism, prolonged severe haemodynamic disturbance may be the most important factor. Patients who deteriorated on medical treatment usually had pulmonary embolectomy, although in one instance a patient deteriorating on heparin has been treated satisfactorily with streptokinase. Our present indications for pulmonary embolectomy include patients deteriorating on medical treatment, those in whom streptokinase is contraindicated, and those who are so ill that the delay in achieving a haemodynamic response is unacceptable.

Because there was no mortality in either treatment group, no conclusion can be made on this aspect. Definite recurrence of pulmonary embolism occurred in only one patient one week after treatment with heparin had been started, so that it is impossible to compare heparin and streptokinase from this point of view. Another question remaining to be answered is the variability in response to both heparin and streptokinase and particularly, perhaps, why rare patients on streptokinase who improve clinically fail to show angiographic improvement over a 72-hour period.

REFERENCES

DALEN, J. E., et al. (1969) *New Eng. J. Med.*, **280,** 1194.
DICKIE, K., et al. (1967) *Tex. Rep. Biol. Med.*, **25,** 613.
FRED, H. L., et al. (1966) *J. Amer. Med. Ass.*, **196,** 1137.
GENTON, E. and WOLF, P. S. (1968) *Amer. Heart J.*, **76,** 628.
GORHAM, L. W. (1961) *Arch. Intern. Med.*, **108,** 8 and 189.
HIRSH, J., et al., (1968) *Brit. med. J.*, **4,** 729.
KERR, I. H., et al. (1971) *Brit. J. Radiol.*, **44,** 751.
MILLER, G. A. H., et al. (1969) *Brit. med. J.*, **1,** 812.
MILLER, G. A. H. and SUTTON, G. C. (1970) *Brit. Heart J.*, **32,** 518.
MURPHY, M. L. and BULLOCK, R. T. (1967) *Clin. Res.*, **15,** 348.
SASAHARA, A. A., et al. (1967) *New Eng. J. Med.*, **277,** 1168.
SAUTTER, R. D., et al. (1967) *J. Amer. Med. Ass.*, **202,** 215.
SAUTTER, R. D., et al. (1967) *Dis. Chest*, **52,** 825.
SCHOLANDER, P. F. (1947) *J. Biol. Chem.*, **167,** 235.
SUTTON, G. C., et al. (1969) *Lancet*, **1,** 271.
SUTTON, G. C. (1970) M. D. Thesis, Cambridge University.
TOW, D. G., et al. (1967) *New Eng. J. Med.*, **277,** 1161.
Urokinase Pulmonary Embolism Trial. Phase I Results. A Co-operative Study. (1970) *J. Amer. Ass.*, **214,** 2163.
ZIJLSTRA, W. G. and MOOK, G. A. (1962). *Medical Reflection Photometry*. Assen. Netherlands.

17 NHLI Urokinase Pulmonary Embolism Trial: Phase I Results of a Controlled Study

A. A. Sasahara, J. S. Belko, G. V. R. K. Sharma, K. M. McIntyre, R. L. Morse and T. M. Hyers

INTRODUCTION

Despite significant advances in diagnostic methodology for pulmonary embolism, there has been a disparate lag in the development of and application of newer and better forms of therapy. Thrombolytic drugs offer great promise of bridging this gap (Sherry, 1968).

From fundamental investigations of clot dissolution in the laboratory (Fig. 17.1), two thrombolytic agents have emerged which appear to have broad applicability in the treatment of thromboembolic disorder. Streptokinase has been used extensively by a number of investigators (Verstraete et al., 1963; Browse and James, 1964; Hirsh et al., 1970), but until recently, its pyrogenicity and antigenicity have limited its use in the United States (Fletcher, 1962; Sherry, 1968). Instead, the newly formed Committee on Thrombolytic Agents of the National Heart and Lung Institute, in 1964, focused its attention on urokinase, the naturally-occurring plasminogen activator present in human urine. Extensive investigations have shown urokinase to be identical, or nearly so, with the plasminogen activators released from human tissues (von Kaulla and Swan, 1958; Smyrniotis et al., 1959; Celander and Guest, 1960). Several important virtues characterise urokinase as a near-optimal lytic agent: it is not antigenic, being of human origin; it is not pyrogenic, having been purified sufficiently to remove contaminants, and its use does not require individualisation of dosage or cautious laboratory control. Its main disadvantage, currently, is its prohibitive cost of production. Streptokinase on the other hand, is antigenic, being a foreign protein of bacterial origin; it is pyrogenic, though improved methods of purification have minimised febrile reactions, and it requires some individualisation of dosage and stricter laboratory control (Editorial, 1967).

From preliminary trials in this country, the feasibility of using urokinase in clinical pulmonary embolism was established (Sasahara *et al.*, 1967; Sautter *et al.*, 1967; Tow *et al.*, 1967). Observations on the ease of administration, dosage and duration of drug infusion, safety and laboratory monitoring were made in a spectrum of

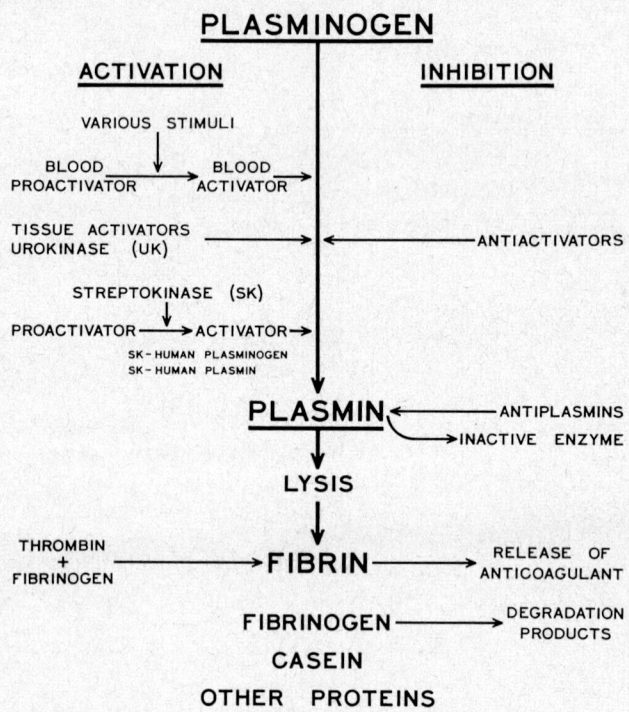

FIG. 17.1. This flow chart of the fibrinolytic process shows the site of action of urokinase and streptokinase.

patients with mild to severe pulmonary embolism. In addition, dramatic dissolution of thromboemboli, with restoration of normal cardiac and pulmonary circulatory dynamics, was noted in some patients. Consequently, the NHLI established a cooperative multi-institutional (14 medical centres) study which was rigidly controlled to compare the results of urokinase followed by heparin therapy with the use of heparin alone. The study, randomised and modified double-blind in design, was directed towards observing differences in the rate and degree of clot resolution in the pulmonary circulation of patients admitted to the trial. The methods used to assess these changes included control and post-infusion pulmonary angiography, control and post-infusion haemodynamic measurements and serial perfusion lung scanning. In addition, other clinical and laboratory abnormalities due to pulmonary embolism were observed for differences in rate of change towards normal in the treatment groups. In view of the relatively low mortality rate of conventionally-treated patients, it was not anticipated that a sample size necessary to demonstrate differences in clot resolution would be adequate to demonstrate differences in mortality during the acute phase of pulmonary embolism. Nor was it felt certain that an accurate comparison of mortality frequency in the two treatment groups could be made in the follow-up period since therapy could not be controlled for such long periods of time. However, clinical assessment and lung scans have been made at 3-, 6- and 12-month follow-ups.

This report is based on the official publication of the NHLI Urokinase Pulmonary Embolism Trial which appeared in the Journal of the American Medical Association (1970).

MATERIALS AND METHODS

Sixteen hospitals, from 14 medical centres, participated in the trial, from October, 1968 to August, 1970. Criteria for eligibility included (1) clinical history of pulmonary embolism within 5 days of anticipated therapy; (2) abnormal lung scan compatible with pulmonary embolism; (3) positive identification of pulmonary embolism by selective angiography; (4) no bleeding diathesis and (5) signed informed consent by the patient. Excluded were those patients with recent operations, recent cerebral vascular accidents and any contraindication to anticoagulant or thrombolytic therapy. All investigators followed a Manual of Operations which was strictly implemented. Procedures, methodology and techniques were all standardised in the 16 institutions. Pre- and post-infusion studies included lung scans, pulmonary angiograms, right heart and pulmonary artery pressures, Fick cardiac outputs, systemic arterial pressures, arterial blood gases and biochemical tests.

Patients receiving urokinase were given a loading dose of 2000 CTA (Committee on Thrombolytic Agents) units/lb body weight, followed by a sustaining dose of 2000 CTA units/lb/hour for 12 hours. Heparin treated patients received a loading dose of 75 units/lb body weight followed by 10 units/lb/hour for 12 hours. After termination of the 12 hour infusion, all patients received heparin intravenously for 5 or more days, followed by oral anticoagulants. Long-term observations included interval history, physical examination and lung scanning at 3-, 6- and 12-month intervals.

Statistical significance was established by using a more conservative method than the conventional 'p' value. Therefore, 'critical ratios' (treatment differences/standard error) were used, 2·5 being of borderline significance and 3·0 being of full significance.

RESULTS

One hundred and sixty patients were admitted, randomised and treated: 78 received heparin and 82 received urokinase followed by

TABLE 17.1

UPET: PATIENT POPULATION

		Heparin	*Urokinase*	*Total*
Total		78	82	160
Sex	Male	45	47	92
	Female	33	35	68
Age	< 50	35	46	81
	> 50	43	36	79
CHF	(clinical)	27	29	56
Angio Severity	Minimal	16	11	27
	Moderate	24	19	43
	Severe	17	26	43
Class	I-S	35	33	68
	I-M	38	40	78
	II-S	1	2	3
	II-M	4	7	11

heparin. Table 17.1 describes the patient population which was matched reasonably well except that the urokinase group tended to be younger and had greater occlusion shown by angiography.

Class I patients had no hypotension while Class II patients did, their systolic pressures being less than 80 mm Hg for at least 10 minutes, and accompanied by appropriate clinical findings of hypotension. 'S' and 'M' refer to angiographic estimate of pulmonary vascular obstruction: 'S' (submassive) involving at least 1 segmental artery and 'M' (massive) involving 2 or more lobar arteries. Except for the massive category and age, the 2 treatment groups were quite comparable.

FIBRINOLYTIC ACTIVITY

The biochemical data concerning lytic control are listed in Table 17.2.

No significant changes in plasminogen or fibrinogen levels were noted in the heparin-treated group, whereas in the urokinase-treated group, plasminogen was reduced 72 per cent and fibrinogen 48 per cent from the control values. Whole blood euglobulin lysis

TABLE 17.2

MEANS OF PRE- AND POST-INFUSION LEVELS

	Heparin mean (S.D.)	Urokinase mean (S.D.)
Plasminogen (CTA Units/ml)		
Pre-	2·17 (0·57)	2·12 (0·59)
Post-	2·24 (0·64)	0·60 (0·42)
Δ	+ 0·07 (0·32)	− 1·52 (0·64)
Fibrinogen (mg%)		
Pre-	493 (159)	515 (200)
Post-	529 (167)	268 (138)
Δ	+ 36 (78)	− 248 (174)
WBELT (minutes)		
Pre-	−	200 (168)
2 hrs.	−	32 (63)
6 hrs.	−	19 (42)
12 hrs.	−	16 (19)

times (WBELT) showed active lysis at 2 hours which was maintained throughout the infusion of urokinase. Some variability did exist among individual patients, but overall, 85 per cent of the patients on urokinase had a good biochemical response to the drug.

PULMONARY ANGIOGRAMS

All angiograms were interpreted independently by an 'expert panel' who had no knowledge of the treatment assignment (Figs. 17.2, 17.3). Methods of analyses were developed, both subjective and objective, which permitted quantification of the perfusion defect. Fig. 17.4 shows the average control or baseline 'severity' of angiographic involvement and the change after drug therapy. Both groups showed 'moderate' involvement which corresponded to approximately 1 lobar artery occlusion. In the heparin-treated group there was minimal improvement after 24 hours, whereas in the urokinase-treated group, the improvement was near 'moderate'. The difference in mean change between the two groups over the

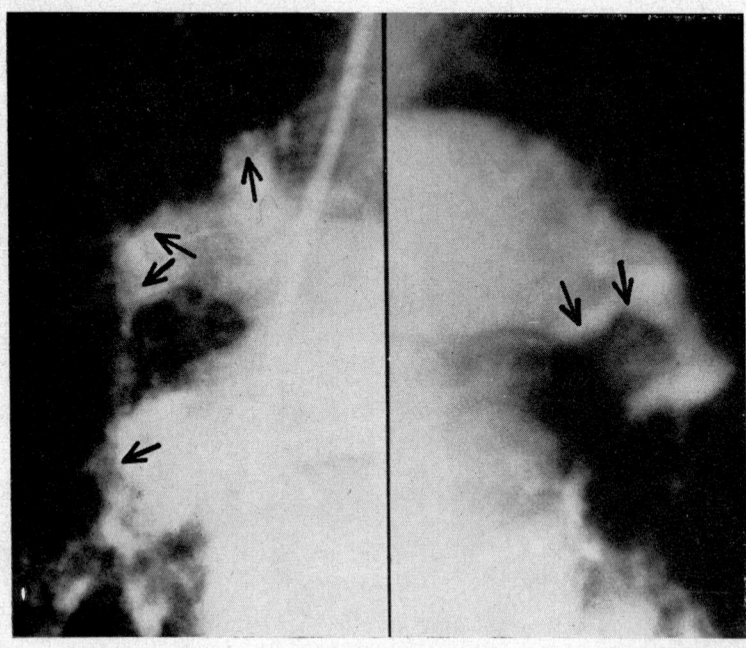

Fig. 17.2. Pre-infusion pulmonary angiogram of a patient with pulmonary embolism. The involvement of the right pulmonary vessels (left panel) includes partial cut-off of right descending lobar pulmonary artery and obstruction of both upper segmental arteries. The left descending lobar artery (right panel) shows intraluminal filling defect and obstruction of segmental vessels.

standard error produced a critical ratio of 5·2 which was highly significant. While few patients showed dramatic improvement, there were many more patients who improved on urokinase than there were on heparin therapy (Figs. 17.5, 17.6). In the heparin-treated group, 5 patients improved 1 class in the post-infusion period, while 24 patients receiving urokinase improved at least 1 class. Four patients improved 2 classes with urokinase, whereas no such improvements were noted with heparin.

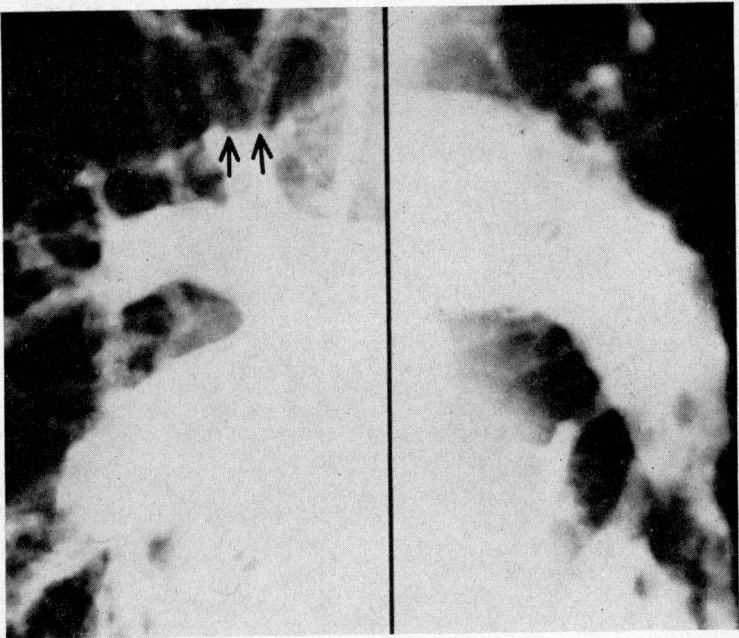

Fig. 17.3. Same patient 24 hours later after urokinase infusion. Note the marked improvement of both right and left pulmonary vessels.

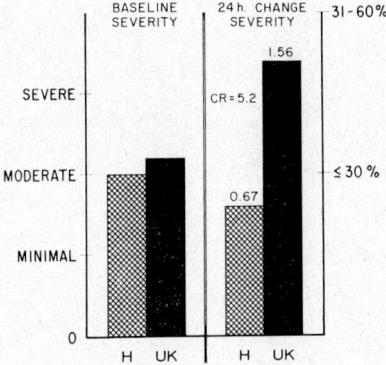

Fig. 17.4. Angiogram baseline and change in the two treatment groups. The urokinase group had slightly more vascular occlusion than the heparin-treated group. The 24-hour change shows greater resolution with urokinase which was highly significant (critical ratio 5.2).

		Pre-Infusion Class				
		I	II	III	IV	TOTAL
Post-Infusion Class	I	0	0	0	0	0
	II	0	16	4	0	20
	III	0	0	20	1	21
	IV	0	0	0	16	16
	TOTAL	0	16	24	17	57

FIG. 17.5. Angiographic severity in the pre- and post-infusion periods reflecting the improvement in clot resolution. Class I is normal; II is minimal angiographic involvement; III is moderate involvement and IV is severe. Note that five patients improved sufficiently with heparin to move up one class in the post-infusion period.

		Pre-Infusion Class				
		I	II	III	IV	TOTAL
Post-Infusion Class	I	1	2	0	0	3
	II	0	9	9	4	22
	III	0	0	10	9	19
	IV	0	0	0	13	13
	TOTAL	1	11	19	26	57

FIG. 17.6. In the urokinase group, 24 patients improved sufficiently to move up at least one class in the post-infusion period. Four patients had greater improvement by angiogram and moved from severe to minimal.

HAEMODYNAMIC MEASUREMENTS

Fig. 17.7 summarises the changes in haemodynamic parameters measured before and after drug therapy. The most frequent abnormalities observed were elevation of right ventricular systolic pressure (greater than 25 mm Hg) and depression of arterial oxygen tension (less than 90 mm Hg) which occurred in 96 per cent and 94 per cent of the patients. Although the average right ventricular systolic pressure was 45 mm Hg, only 15 per cent had systolic pressures greater than 60 mm Hg. Of the 8 parameters listed in Fig. 17.7,

6 showed significant improvement towards normal in the urokinase-treated group while in 2, arterio-venous oxygen difference and cardiac index, no significant difference existed between the two groups. The most significant change occurred in total pulmonary resistance which, because of the wide spread, was expressed as the natural log of the resistance. It was of interest to note that in the 24-hour period, patients treated with heparin showed little if any change in haemodynamics.

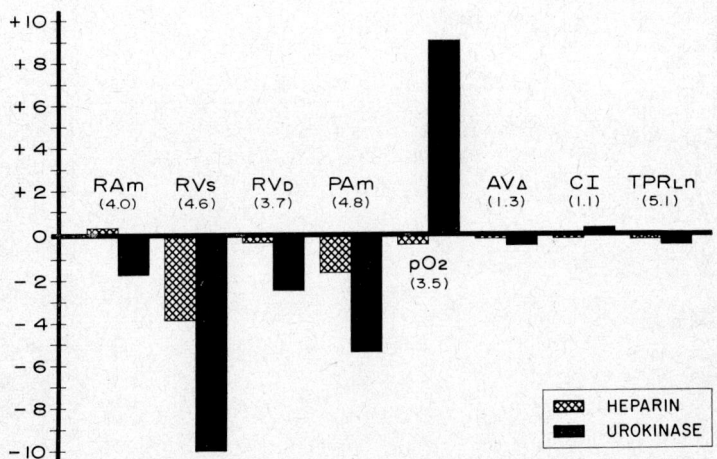

FIG. 17.7. Eight haemodynamic parameters with their mean changes in 24 hours are depicted here for the two groups. The scale is in the appropriate units: mm Hg for pressures and gas tension; volumes per cent for AV differences; litre/min/M^2 for cardiac index and natural logarithms for total pulmonary resistance. The wide range of resistances necessitated using natural logs. The most significant changes were noted in the pulmonary resistance. Only arterio-venous difference and cardiac index were not significantly different.

LUNG SCANNING

Lung scans were also evaluated independently by an expert panel who had no knowledge of patient treatment. The scans were assessed by visual techniques and the perfusion deficits were expressed as a percentage of total normal perfusion of both lungs. The mean baseline or control deficit in both groups was approximately 25 per cent which corresponds to a perfusion defect of one-half of one lung. The percentage of the initial lesion which resolved during the first 24 hours was 8·1 per cent in the heparin-treated group and 22·1 per cent in the urokinase-treated group (Fig. 17.8). This is a significant difference which parallels the improvement noted in the angiograms and haemodynamic data. At 5 days and at 14 days, however, there was no significant difference in the percentage resolution. In contrast, the greatest improvement during the 24-hour and subsequent periods occurred in the I-M (massive without shock) group treated with urokinase which showed greater resolution until the thirteenth and fourteenth day, at which time no significant differences were noted. Although not all patients in Class II-M (massive with shock) had scans performed, 4 treated with urokinase showed percentage resolution ranging from 33·4–68·6 per cent, while the only patient in this category receiving heparin showed a percentage resolution of 6·2 per cent.

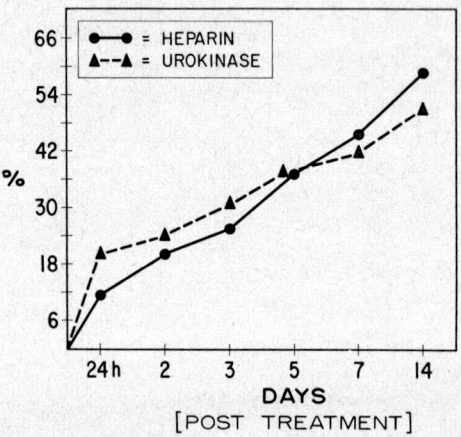

FIG. 17.8. Mean per cent resolution for both groups estimated by scans. Note the small but significant improvement in scan resolution in the first 24 hours, which diminished by the fifth day.

COMPLICATIONS OF THERAPY

No febrile, anaphylactic or other untoward reactions were noted with urokinase administration. Selected tests of liver function did not show any change. The most common complication noted in both groups of patients was overt bleeding or unexplained falls in haematocrit. Twenty-one patients (27 per cent) in the heparin-treated group and 36 patients (44 per cent) in the urokinase-treated group had bleeding complications which were classified as moderate (blood loss of 500–1500 ml; haematocrit fall of 5–10 per cent; blood transfusion of two units or less) or severe (exceeding the moderate criteria) (Table 17.3).

The majority of patients in the urokinase-treated group who bled did so in the early period, i.e., within the first 24 hours while uro-

TABLE 17.3
UPET: HAEMORRHAGIC COMPLICATIONS

		Heparin	Urokinase
Total		21 (27%)	36 (44%)
Early	Moderate	4	15
	Severe	5	13
Late	Moderate	6	0
	Severe	6	8

kinase was being infused. Thereafter, there was no increase in bleeding compared to the heparin-treated group. In the heparin group, about the same number bled early as they did late. It is of interest to note that during the late period (after 24 hours), although the numbers bleeding in each treatment group were not significantly different, the urokinase-treated group had more extensive bleeding. Further analysis of bleeding (Table 17.4) shows that the increased frequency of bleeding in patients receiving urokinase therapy was associated with sites of invasive procedures, i.e., cutdown sites for pulmonary arterial catheter insertion and arterial puncture sites.

TABLE 17.4
UPET: HAEMORRHAGIC COMPLICATIONS

	Heparin	Urokinase
Cutdown	6	20
moderate	2	13
severe	4	7
Spontaneous	15	16
moderate	7	2
severe	8	14
HCT Falls (Idiopathic)	20 (26%)	20 (24%)
moderate	19	15
severe	1	5

Spontaneous haemorrhage, on the other hand, occurred with equal frequency in both groups; but again, when it did occur, bleeding tended to be severe, as compared to the heparin-treated group which had equal numbers in the moderate and severe categories. In both treatment groups, bleeding from venous cutdown sites was much more troublesome than arterial sites. It was difficult, in many instances, to maintain perfect haemostasis around the indwelling angiographic catheter, as well as to maintain the optimal amount of pressure at other invasive sites. In many patients, scattered haematoma discolouration in the arm with the angiographic catheter was not uncommon. Overt oozing from the invasive sites was particularly troublesome in the obese patient. Unexplained haematocrit falls occurred with the same frequency in both groups. They were rarely severe and did not necessitate transfusion. In all likelihood, they were associated with frequent venepunctures necessary for the performance of all biochemical tests required in this trial.

TABLE 17.5

UPET: OTHER COMPLICATIONS

	Heparin	Urokinase
PE (recurrent)	15	11
definite	2	3
probable	13	8
Acute MI	1	0
IVC Procedures	9	3
Embolectomy	0	0
Death	7	6
I-S : 4/68 (5·9%)		
I-M : 4/78 (5·1%)		
II-S : 3/3 (100%)		
II-M : 2/11 (18·2%)		

Recurrence of pulmonary embolism during the first two weeks occurred in 15 patients treated with heparin and 11 patients treated with urokinase (Table 17.5).

Recurrence was considered proved if both lung scan evidence and clinical evidence were obtained. An episode was probable if only one of these was obtained. While recurrences were generally well tolerated, one was fatal for a patient who had received urokinase 10 days before.

In the two-week observation period, seven patients in the heparin-treated group and six in the urokinase-treated group died. Six of the heparin group died from cardiorespiratory arrest and the seventh from complicating myocardial infarction. Of the six in the urokinase group, three died from cardiorespiratory arrest, one from recurrent pulmonary embolism, one from massive cerebral haemorrhage (stroke one month previously) and the last from pneumonia. Further analysis of mortality shows that the great majority of patients in Class I, whether massive or submassive, survived the embolic insult.

In addition, only two of 11 patients in shock with massive embolism succumbed, whereas all three patients in shock with submassive embolism as judged by angiography, succumbed. The latter three patients were critically ill with cardiopulmonary compromise prior to embolisation and deteriorated rapidly with 'sublethal' amounts of pulmonary vascular occlusion. The overall mortality of the trial was 8·1 per cent.

DISCUSSION

This first phase of the NHLI study of thrombolytic therapy was terminated when data from the three parameters used in end-point analysis showed significant differences in treatment improvement with urokinase in comparison to heparin therapy. Angiography, which was the most sensitive indicator in this study showed significantly greater clot resolution with urokinase; haemodynamic parameters, next in sensitivity, showed significantly greater return towards normal with urokinase, and finally lung scans, after 160 patients were admitted to the trial, showed significantly greater perfusion return with urokinase.

The data have therapeutic implications, particularly for patients who suffered massive or near-massive embolism, since this group appeared to show the greatest response to urokinase treatment. It is also of interest to note that during the trial, 11 patients were not entered into the trial because of massive embolism. All were subjected to pulmonary embolectomy with an operative mortality of 73 per cent. Although this group may not be comparable to the Class II-M patients, the striking difference in mortality (73 per cent versus 18 per cent) suggests that pulmonary embolectomy may not be the preferred treatment in most patients with shock and massive embolism. Despite the fact that no differences in mortality were demonstrated in this 160 patient study, no conclusion can be drawn in relationship to drug treatment and mortality. It is of interest, however, to speculate on the basis of the data currently available. Of the seven deaths in the heparin-treated group, six died from cardiorespiratory failure whereas only three of the six in the urokinase group died of cardiorespiratory failure. In view of the significant early improvement in haemodynamic parameters associated with greater clot resolution by angiography and greater perfusion by lung scan in urokinase patients, it seems reasonable to expect fewer patients to succumb from cardiorespiratory failure with urokinase therapy. Perhaps in a larger series, this difference in mortality may become evident. The complete evaluation of the benefits of thrombolytic therapy was also hampered by the fact that multiple invasive procedures, not ordinarily done in similar clinical situations, contributed heavily to morbidity in the form of overt bleeding. Although the incidence of spontaneous bleeding was the same in both treatment groups, a clear assessment of the safety of the drug was not possible in this trial.

Although the results were unequivocal in fulfilling the aim of the trial, several important questions remain unanswered: would a longer duration of therapy have resulted in more dramatic resolutions of thromboemboli, both in the lungs and in the venous formation sites, and could greater thrombolysis by increased infusion time be achieved without increasing morbidity and mortality? The current Phase II Trial is seeking answers to these questions, as well as to compare the efficacy of streptokinase, currently more available, to urokinase.

ACKNOWLEDGEMENT

We would like to acknowledge the other principal investigators from the many institutions involved in this trial: Dr. John R. Blackmon (University of Washington); Dr. Richard D. Sautter (Marshfield Clinic Foundation); Dr. Henry N. Wagner, Jr. (Johns Hopkins Medical Institutions); Dr. Noble O. Fowler (Cincinnati General Hospital); Dr. Edward Genton (University of Colorado Medical Centre); Dr. Joseph V. Messer (Boston City Hospital); Dr. Donald Silver (Duke University Medical Centre); Dr. Park W. Willis III (University of Michigan Medical Centre); Dr. James E. Dalen (Peter Bent Brigham Hospital); Dr. Nanette K. Wenger (Emory University School of Medicine); Dr. Frank J. Hildner (Mount Sinai Hospital of Greater Miami); Dr. Robert N. Cooley (University of Texas Medical Branch); Dr. Robert M. Stanzler (Cook County Hospital).

We also wish to acknowledge the helpful guidance of Dr. Sol Sherry, Chairman, Policy Board; Dr. James M. Stengle, Director National Blood Resource Branch, National Heart and Lung Institute and Dr. Peter N. Walsh, former Liaison Officer, UPET Project, National Heart and Lung Institute.

We are also indebted to the following members of our local UPET team who have been available on a 24-hour basis: Scan Team: Robert G. Simpson, Paul F. Godin and Curtis E. Wrenn; Angiographic Team: Lucy Massa and Leo Barron; Blood Analysis Team: Virginia A. Burleson, Helen Guilford and Barbara Roggeveen, and Biochemical Team: James R. Wrenn. Finally, we are grateful to Miss Donna Caroselli for invaluable editorial assistance.

REFERENCES

BROWSE, N. L. and JAMES, D. C. O. (1964) *Lancet*, **2**, 1039.
CELANDER, D. R. and GUEST, M. M. (1960) *Amer. J. Cardiol.*, **6**, 409.
FLETCHER, A. P. et al. (1962) *Amer. J. Med.*, **33**, 738.
HIRSH, J. et al. (1970) *Blood*, **35**, 341.
VON KAULLA, K. N. and SWAN, H. (1958) *J. Thoracic Surg.*, **36**, 519.
SASAHARA, A. A. et al. (1967) *New Engl. J. Med.*, **277**, 1168.
SAUTTER, R. D. et al. (1967) *J. Amer. Med. Ass.*, **202**, 215.
SHERRY, S. (1968) *Ann. Rev. Med.*, **19**, 247.
SMYRNIOTIS, F. E. et al. (1959) *Thromb. et Diath. Haemorrh.*, **3**, 257.
TOW, D. E. et al. (1967) *New Engl. J. Med.*, **277**, 1161.
UROKINASE EDITORIAL (1967) *New Engl. M. Med.*, **277**, 203.
UROKINASE PULMONARY EMBOLISM TRIAL, (1970) *J. Amer. Med. Ass.*, **214**, 2163.
VERSTRAETE, M. et al. (1963) *Brit. med. J.*, **1**, 1499.

PART IV
SURGICAL TREATMENT

18 Embolectomy and Pulmonary Embolism: Criteria for Surgery

P. A. Cullum, V. V. Kakkar, A. M. Macarthur, S. Oram and E. B. Raftery

INTRODUCTION

The availability of thrombolytic agents, such as streptokinase and urokinase, is rapidly altering the approach to the treatment of acute massive pulmonary embolism. As a result the indications for operative intervention have narrowed considerably and the number of patients referred for surgery has diminished. Nevertheless, the need still exists for embolectomy in the management of the critically ill patient. Indeed, there is no certain method of predicting the likelihood of death or survival in those patients treated by thrombolysis. It would clarify the position if cases could be identified in which the obstructing embolus was not responsive and invariably proved fatal before lysis was completed, so that they might proceed to surgery without delay.

We report here the clinical and angiographic appearances of 22 patients which we have found helpful in the selection of cases for thrombolysis or surgery.

MATERIALS AND METHODS

SELECTION OF PATIENTS

The patients were seen over a five-year period. The first nine patients were seen before streptokinase became available, and the last 13 represent a combined medical and surgical approach.

PULMONARY ANGIOGRAPHY

A No. 8 Lehman catheter was passed from an arm vein to the pulmonary artery and 30–40 ml of 75 per cent sodium metrizoate was injected into the pulmonary artery by means of a pressure injector (100 lb per sq in) and single-plane (anteroposterior) serial arteriograms were obtained using a synchronised automatic film changer.

The angiographic appearances were assessed by an index of severity (Sutton *et al.*, page 181) and by estimation of the reduction of peripheral perfusion. This latter index is an assessment of the number of opacified vessels reaching the periphery of the lung fields, gauged during an early phase of angiography, when unoccluded vessels are seen to have filled normally.

ADMINISTRATION OF STREPTOKINASE

Streptokinase (Kabikinase) was given by continuous infusion; in three patients it was administered through the pulmonary arterial catheter, while in the remainder a peripheral vein was used. A 'loading dose' of 500,000 units was given over the first 30 minutes; this was followed by a maintenance dose of 150,000 units per hour.

PULMONARY EMBOLECTOMY

Cardiopulmonary bypass was established in the usual manner, using a median sternotomy incision, and right atrial to ascending aortic cannulation (Paneth *et al.*, page 223). A no-blood prime was preferred so that there was no delay waiting for blood to be cross-matched, and any deficit in the post-operative haematacrit was corrected by transfusion later. Where patients were severely hypotensive, and in order to avoid cardiac arrest during and after induction of anaesthesia, femoral arterial cannulation was performed under a local anaesthetic on the operating table so that only right atrial cannulation was required to establish cardiopulmonary bypass. Embolectomy was performed after fibrillating the heart, cross-clamping the great vessels and opening the main pulmonary artery with a longitudinal incision. After removal of the main emboli, the last clots were extracted under direct vision, using a Desjardin forceps, while the lungs were gently expanded by positive pressure ventilation. Bypass time was usually less than 30 minutes.

RESULTS

Nine patients received streptokinase and of these, two died. Thirteen patients underwent surgery and of these, four died. The clinical and angiographic appearances were analysed in detail to see what factors, if any, were common to those who did not survive.

COMPARISON OF CLINICAL STATUS

No patient had a previous history of cardio-respiratory disease. The average age of the streptokinase patients was 46 years, (37–62) and of the operated patients 48 years, (26–68). There were seven males in the streptokinase group and only five in the operated group. No patient had had an acute history of more than 48 hours; in 16 this was 24 hours or less. The mean systolic blood pressure (defined as the cuff pressure taken at the time of decision to proceed to angiography or surgery) was significantly higher in those patients receiving streptokinase ($P < 0.001$), reflecting the clinical approach to the problem. No patient went to surgery who did not appear to be critically ill. Cardiac arrest occurred prior to treatment in one streptokinase patient and six times in four patients proceeding to

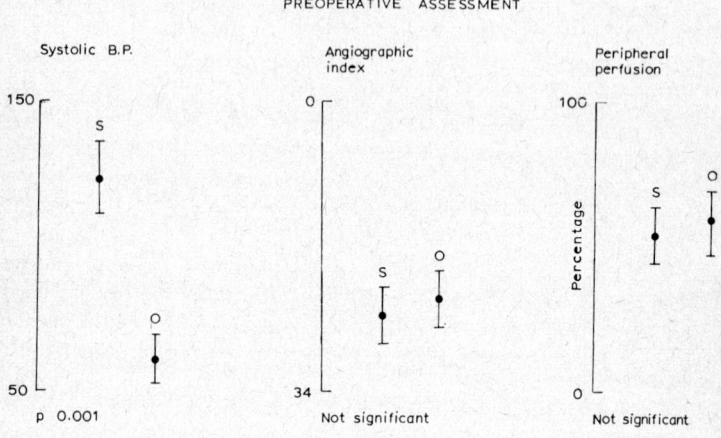

Fig. 18.1. Pre-operative assessment.

surgery. However, there was no significant difference in the angiographic index of severity or peripheral perfusion in those patients having angiography between the streptokinase group and the operated group (Fig. 18.1).

RELATIONSHIP OF MEAN SYSTOLIC BLOOD PRESSURE TO ANGIOGRAPHIC APPEARANCES

The mean systolic blood pressure was compared with that of 17 patients who had had angiography, to see what relationship, if any, existed between it and the angiographic index of severity, as well as the peripheral perfusion. Although patients with less severe angiographic appearances had near-normal or normal systolic blood pressures, and those with severe changes were hypotensive, a linear relationship was not shown. Indeed, in those patients with a systolic blood pressure between 110 and 90 there was considerable variation (Fig. 18.2).

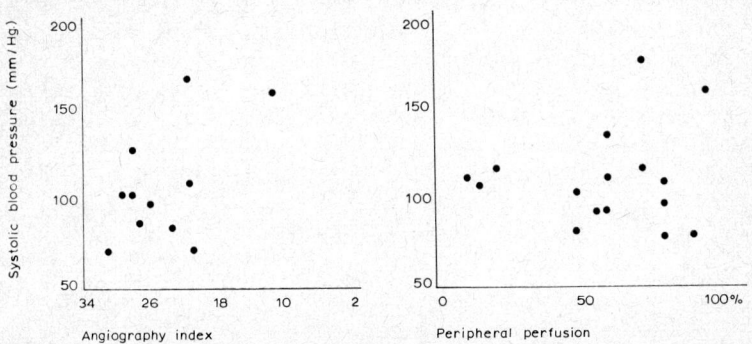

FIG. 18.2. Relationship of mean systolic pressure to angiographic appearances.

OPERATIVE MORTALITY

Four patients (31 per cent) of those operated upon died, two from recurrent, acute massive pulmonary embolism. Comparison of the mean systolic blood pressure, angiographic index of severity and the peripheral perfusion between survivors and non-survivors did not reveal a significant difference in the two sub-groups, although the non-survivors tended to have an improved systolic blood pressure and angiographic appearance (Fig. 18.3).

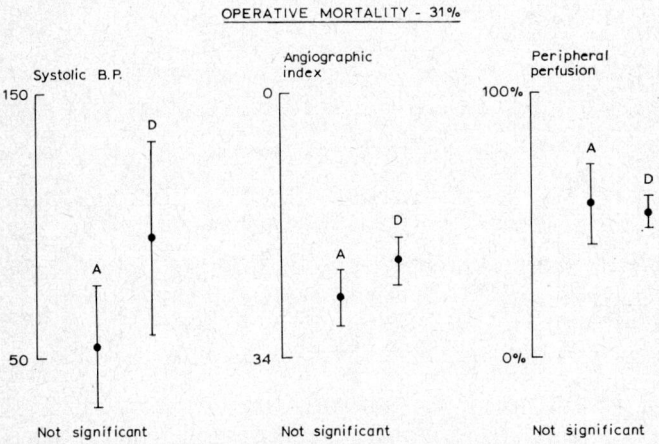

FIG. 18.3. Operative mortality.

STREPTOKINASE MORTALITY

Two female patients, aged 62 and 37 years respectively, died during streptokinase therapy from cardiac arrest. Neither patient was considered ill enough for surgery at the time of decision. Again there was no significant difference between the mean systolic blood pressure and angiographic index of severity between survivors and non-survivors, although the non-survivors had a systolic blood pressure of 105 and 110 mm Hg with an angiographic index of severity of 29/34 and 30/34 points respectively. However, the duration of symptoms in both patients was the least in the group (18 and 4 hours).

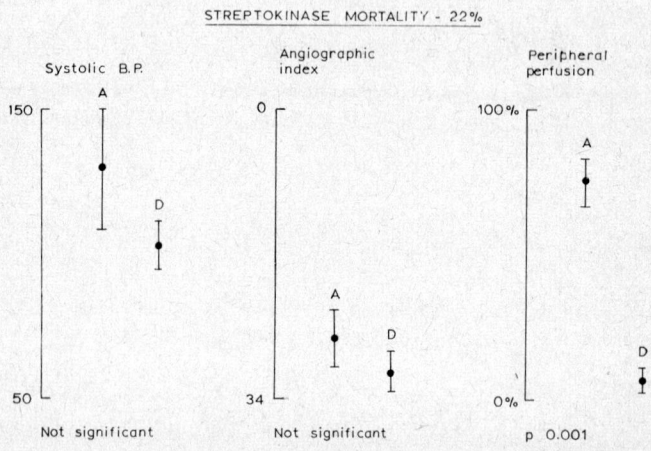

FIG. 18.4. Streptokinase mortality.

The peripheral perfusion had been reduced by more than 75 per cent in each patient, and this was highly significant ($p < 0.001$) when compared with the surviving patients (Figs. 18.4, 18.5, 18.6).

DISCUSSION

The place of streptokinase in the treatment of pulmonary embolism has not yet been defined. It is of extreme importance to choose the correct treatment for patients with major embolism who survive the acute episode. Embolectomy, although it may be life-saving, carries a high mortality and morbidity; and cannot be recommended for every patient with major embolism. Unfortunately, the same is also true of streptokinase therapy, and although it has been shown to be effective it has disadvantages in patients who are critically ill

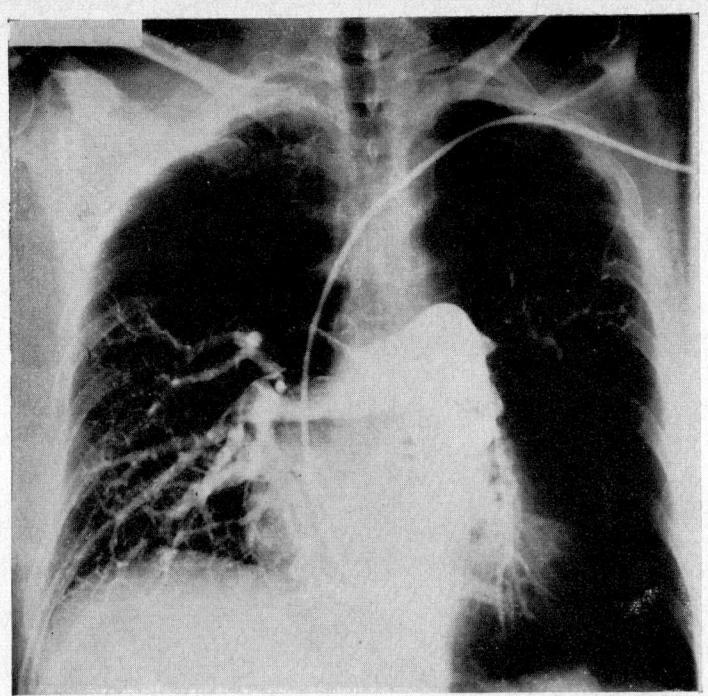
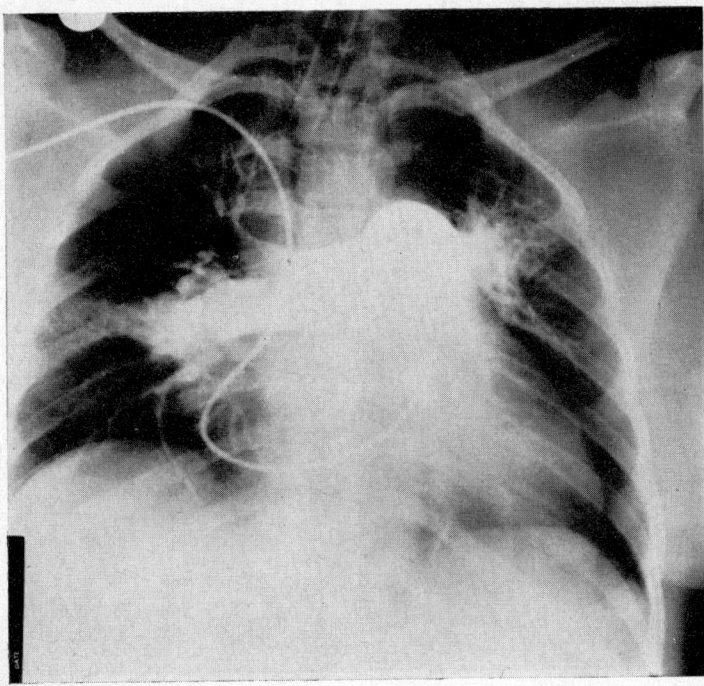

Fig. 18.5. Angiographic appearances before and after treatment.

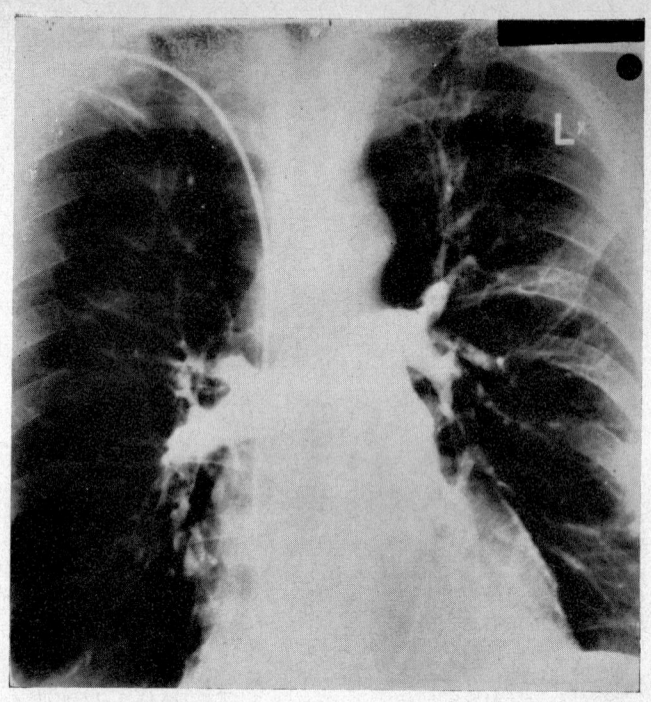
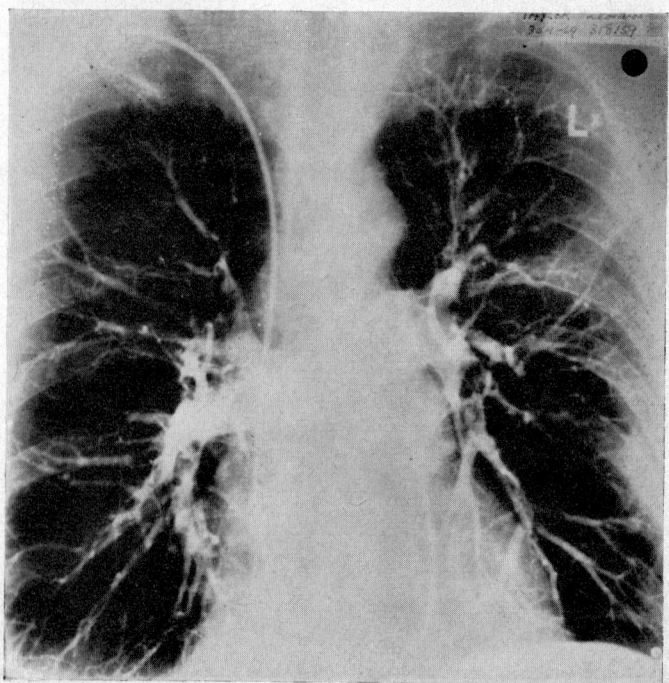

Fig. 18,6. Angiographic appearances before and after treatment.

with a poor respiratory reserve. The most important objective is to remove the embolus before cardiac decompensation; dissolution with streptokinase takes time. Furthermore, streptokinase does not always dissolve thrombi.

Studies in patients with extensive deep vein thrombosis using streptokinase have shown a poor result when the thrombus is more than 72 hours old and when it completely occludes the lumen. Many pulmonary emboli may be more than 72 hours duration when first diagnosed and are not suitable for thrombolytic therapy.

Although the local perfusion of streptokinase over a period of 72 hours may dissolve peripheral emboli, in order to deal effectively with the peripheral thrombus a longer infusion of up to seven days is often necessary. Failure to take into consideration this aspect of treatment can result in rethrombosis of the peripheral veins and repeated pulmonary embolism.

There is clear evidence that some patients benefit from streptokinase infusion; it is therefore important to define which patients should be treated by streptokinase and which should proceed to surgery. It has been suggested that, if a patient is shocked, with a systolic blood pressure of less than 100 mm Hg, a raised central venous pressure and evidence of renal failure, then surgery is indicated. In our studies, the mean systolic blood pressure was significantly lower in those patients proceeding to operation than in those treated by streptokinase therapy, reflecting the clinical approach to the problem. There was no difference between the two groups when a comparison was made of the angiographic appearances, neither was there a linear relationship between the mean systolic blood pressure and the angiographic appearances when these were plotted against each other. Clearly, factors such as age, co-existing cardio-respiratory disease, duration and severity of symptoms, and of treatment, play their separate parts in the natural history of the disease.

That there were no significant differences between the mean systolic blood pressure and the angiographic appearances in the survivors and non-survivors in the operated group would indicate that the cause of death was neither a result of massive embolism, nor directly related to embolectomy, but rather due to the complications of cardiac surgery. In contrast, both the systolic blood pressure and the angiographic index of severity was lower in the non-survivors of streptokinase treated patients, who died before thrombolysis was effective. However, no significant difference existed between the general condition of those patients who died and those who survived, and the absence of clinical shock was an important factor in favour of thrombolytic therapy. Similarly a previous report has indicated that the electrocardiogram and haemodynamic investigations during angiography were also of no value in distinguishing between those patients who died and those who survived.

The only differences were in the pulmonary angiograms. In each patient who survived, angiography showed extensive emboli but the peripheral perfusion of the lungs was good. In contrast, the angiograms of the patients who died showed massive emboli in the major vessels, and the peripheral perfusion of the lungs was poor. Both the

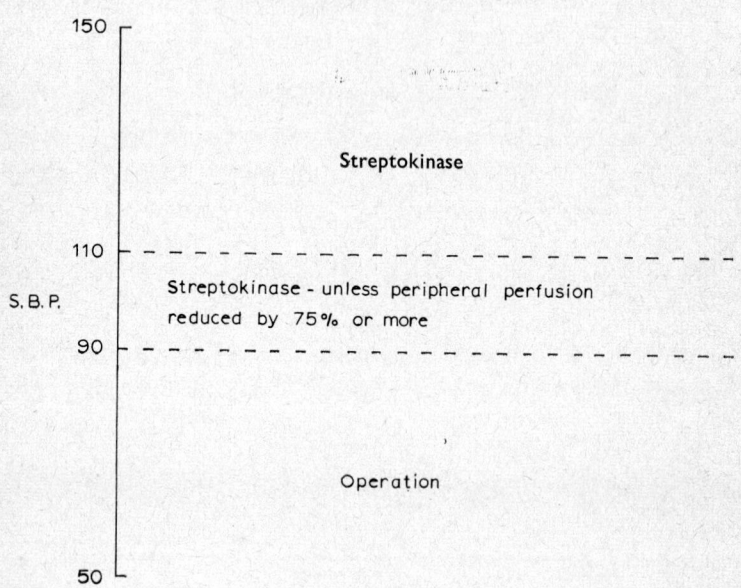

Fig. 18.7. Guidelines for treatment.

patients who died had had their emboli for less than 18 hours, whereas the remainder had had symptoms for 24 hours or more. This suggests that there may be a functional problem associated with pulmonary blood flow which is best indicated by a measurement of the peripheral lung perfusion seen angiographically, and that, at the time of decision, their functional reserve was very low although their clinical appearances did not suggest this. It would seem that the amount of peripheral perfusion seen angiographically is the best indication of functional reserve; thus where the peripheral perfusion is reduced by 75 per cent the patient should be referred to surgery and not treated by thrombolytic therapy (Fig. 18.7).

SUMMARY

Twenty-two patients with acute massive pulmonary embolism were treated either by streptokinase or embolectomy; 6 or 27 per cent died. Clinical and angiographic findings show that a measurement of the peripheral perfusion after pulmonary angiography is the single most important investigation in selecting those patients most likely to benefit from streptokinase therapy.

19 Surgical Treatment of Pulmonary Embolism
M. Paneth

Interest in massive pulmonary embolism at the Brompton Hospital arose from a number of fatalities associated with the performance of the standard Trendelenberg procedure.

The effect of impaction of an embolus in the pulmonary arterial tree is purely mechanical. Thus, experimental obstruction of the

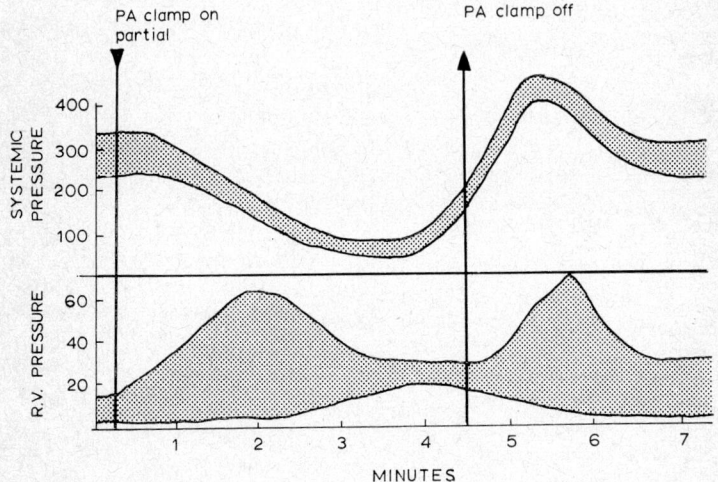

FIG. 19.1. Systemic and right ventricular pressures after partially clamping the pulmonary artery.

pulmonary artery, sufficient to lower systemic pressure, causes a convulsive effort of the right ventricle for about two minutes, followed by a rise in diastolic pressure. The process is repeatable; the composite result from several experiments is shown in Fig. 19.1. No evidence of airway obstruction or vascular spasm due to release of serotonin or other vasoactive substances has been found.

It is important to make a correct diagnosis before instituting treatment—medical or surgical. However, some patients have to be treated on the basis of a presumptive clinical diagnosis, because they are too ill to undergo pulmonary angiography.

An analysis of the first 50 cases of massive pulmonary embolism which have been studied at the Brompton Hospital for predisposing factors showed that recent surgery had been performed in two-thirds (Table 19.1).

TABLE 19.1

PREDISPOSING FACTORS

Recent surgery	33 (66%)
Deep venous thrombosis alone	4 (8%)
Recent surgery and oral contraceptives	3 (6%)
Oral contraceptives alone	3 (6%)
Pregnancy	2 (4%)
Steroid therapy	1 (2%)
Bed rest (prolapsed disc)	1 (2%)
Mitral stenosis	1 (2%)
Recent myocardial infarction	1 (2%)

Pulmonary embolism presents with 'collapse', possibly cardiac arrest, central chest pain due probably to myocardial ischaemia, and dyspnoea due to diminished cardiac output. The incidence of these factors is given in Table 19.2.

TABLE 19.2

PRESENTING SYMPTOMS—INCIDENCE

Collapse	82%
Dyspnoea	74%
Circulatory arrest	24%
Central chest pain	32%
Pleurisy and/or haemoptysis	20%
Premonitory pleurisy and/or haemoptysis	32%

Thus, the patient prefers to lie down rather than to sit up, and may faint if sat up for examination. Frequently there are minor preceding emboli which may give rise to premonitory pleurisy and/or haemoptysis.

The response to a reduction in cardiac output is sinus tachycardia with a gallop rhythm or an additional heart sound. Elevation of central venous pressure is obvious unless the patient already has been treated with diuretics. Table 19.3 gives data on the frequency with which these and other physical signs were observed.

TABLE 19.3

PHYSICAL SIGNS

Sinus tachycardia	86%
*Blood pressure less than 80 mm Hg systolic	30%
Elevated central venous pressure	82%
Gallop rhythm (left sternal edge)	89%
Central cyanosis	62%
Clinical deep venous thrombosis	32%

*At time of admission—some patients were receiving vasopressor agents.

A confident clinical diagnosis can be made in 90 per cent of cases from these observations. Moreover, a plain chest X-ray is of great value because of the presence of oligaemic zones; a prominent hilar shadow can often be seen (Table 19.4).

TABLE 19.4

PLAIN X-RAY FINDINGS

Feature	Angio (n = 25)	Operation (n = 8)	Total n = 33
Oligaemic zones	25	8	33 (100%)
Hyperaemic zones	10	0	10 (30%)
Prominent hilar shadows	14	5	19 (58%)
Infarct shadow	14	3	17 (51%)
Elevated dome of diaphragm	7	4	11 (33%)
Dilated main pulmonary trunk	3	0	3 (9%)
Not available	13		
Not assessable	3		

Electrocardiographic changes, a wide arterio-venous oxygen difference and an elevation of right ventricular end-diastolic pressure are other features found during cardiac catheterisation.

PULMONARY EMBOLECTOMY

The operative approach for pulmonary embolectomy is by a vertical median sternotomy. If there is no time to institute perfusion, a modified Trendelenberg procedure is carried out. Whereas in the original procedure the outflow tracts were occluded, non-crushing clamps are applied to the inferior vena cava and superior vena cava in that order, and the heart is massaged to empty it. Then, using a side clamp, the pulmonary trunk is opened, and as much

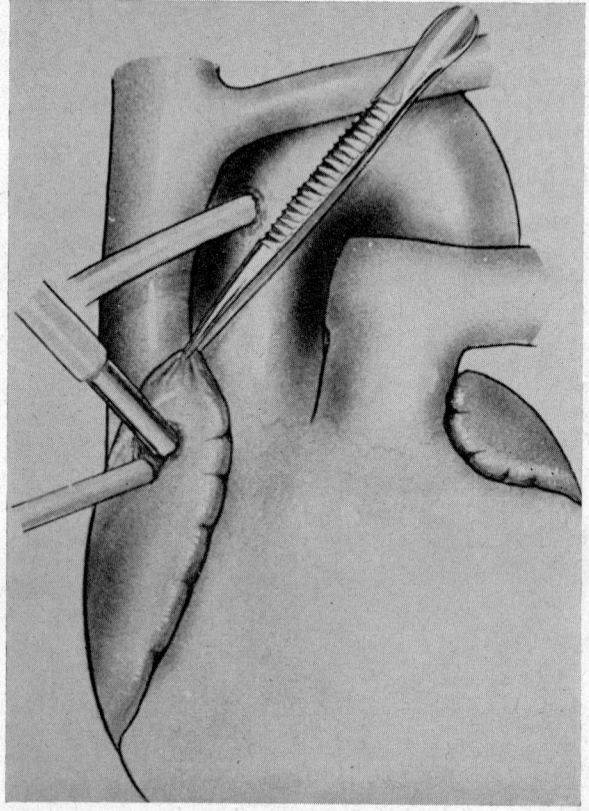

FIG. 19.2. Insertion of bypass cannulae into the root of the aorta and the right auricular appendage.

embolus as possible is sucked out from each branch in turn over a two minute period. During this procedure the circulation is virtually arrested.

The circulation is then restored by clamping the incision in the pulmonary trunk and releasing the superior vena caval clamp, thus allowing slow filling of the heart. By a gradual release of the inferior vena caval clamp, the heart is not overfilled while regaining tone and function. If further emboli are to be extracted, the whole process can be repeated after allowing about 15 minutes for cerebral, coronary and renal perfusion—massaging the heart meanwhile if necessary.

The process of repeated extraction of embolus can clear the pulmonary circulation to a sufficient extent to allow the heart to maintain a satisfactory output unaided.

The better alternative involves bypass with cannulae in the root of the aorta and into the right atrium via its appendage (Fig. 19.2). When these cannulae are connected to the arterial and venous limbs of the bypass circuit, the heart and lungs are totally circumvented. Moreover, the right ventricle is relieved of its overload. Because the aorta is perfused with fully oxygenated blood at the physiological minute volume, the cerebral, coronary and renal flow is restored to normal.

Then the pulmonary trunk is opened by a longitudinal incision and each pulmonary arterial tree is carefully cleared of all visible emboli.

Repeated inflation of the lungs by the anaesthetist massages the lungs and produces retrograde filling of both sides with red blood if all the emboli have been cleared. The incision in the pulmonary trunk can then be closed, followed by loose closure of the pericardium, leaving drainage tubes in situ.

The surgical mortality in ten patients with a history of circulatory arrest has been 80 per cent. However, there was no mortality in patients with this history who were treated thrombolytically (Miller et al., 1971), and with more experience, the overall surgical mortality has fallen to 25 per cent.

Although Gorham (1961) found that two-thirds of patients with pulmonary embolism die in the first two hours, resuscitation by external cardiac massage and the administration of vasopressors should lower this figure. Stabilisation, with a systemic blood pressure above 80 mm Hg without repeated and increasing doses of vasopressors, may not be achieved, and an emergency embolectomy using the modified Trendelenberg procedure may have to be carried out.

If the patient is stable, angiography can be performed to confirm the diagnosis and to assess severity. Under these circumstances, there is a choice between embolectomy with cardiac by-pass or thrombolytic therapy, which has become the first line of attack. If at any time the patient becomes unstable, as shown by a fall in cardiac output, embolectomy with cardiac by-pass can still be performed.

REFERENCES

GORHAM, L. W. (1961) *Arch. Int. Med.*, **108,** 189.
MILLER, G. A. H. *et al.* (1971) *Brit. med. J.*, **2,** 681.

20 Discussions to Parts 3 and 4

Widmer: Because clinical signs are so misleading, objective examination such as phlebography is essential. Thus, our procedure involves at least two phlebograms (before treatment and, on average, five days after the start of treatment).

Of about 160 of our patients, some 12 per cent were treated surgically. Among the remainder we have phlebograms for 73 patients treated with streptokinase and 23 with anticoagulants. The two groups were well matched for sex, age, delay between the onset of the disease and the start of treatment and the interval between initial and follow-up phlebography. All the phlebograms were reviewed by a panel comprising an angiologist, a radiologist and a coagulation expert; all were in ignorance of which treatment was employed.

Ninety-three of these patients had widespread occlusion, involving the femoral and iliac veins—enough to disturb venous return severely. With thrombolytic therapy, 45 per cent of the cases showed a good result, i.e. major veins were re-opened, and another 25 per cent showed a partially successful outcome. One patient deteriorated, however; the proximal two-thirds of the femoral vein became occluded during thrombolysis.

We had no real success with heparin—in only 7 per cent could the veins be visualised.

We have attempted to assess the extent of re-opening of occluded veins. With thrombolytic therapy, only 20–30 per cent success was achieved in the lower leg, about 40 per cent in the femoral vein and about 60 per cent in re-opening of the venous 'star' where the four veins meet. This is an important observation.

Although thrombolysis often is terminated after 72 hours, we have, in 18 of the 73 patients, continued for several days. For example, recanalisation of many occluded veins has been observed within five days, but continuing thrombolysis for two more days has resulted in complete clearance.

In both groups a check for pulmonary embolism was made. The small group of heparin-treated patients had a 4 per cent incidence of non-fatal embolism; the incidence in the streptokinase groups was 4·5 per cent. Fatal embolism did not occur in either group. Thus, there is no increased danger of pulmonary embolism with streptokinase thrombolysis.

We think that treatment with streptokinase may be very useful. Although many regard it as expensive treatment, the cost is probably 40–50 times less than that of the post-thrombotic syndrome.

Johnson: The lung scans from the urokinase pulmonary embolism trial showed that resolution with heparin treatment was much slower than with urokinase, when the embolism was less than 48 hours old. Surprisingly, there was little difference between the treatments with embolism older than 48 hours.

It has been said that LDH and other enzyme changes are useful in the diagnosis of pulmonary embolism. Our findings do not support this.

The pre-treatment levels of FR-antigen were not as high as was anticipated. The normal value is less than 1·0 μg, and for 49 patients, the mean level was $3 \pm 1·7$ μg. In six, however, the mean level was $26·6 \pm 15$ μg.

Using a fibrinolytic assay for urokinase, the mean level for the 12 hour blood sample was 50 units, and the level was relatively uniform at 6, 12 and 18 hours. However, the range between individuals varied widely.

We have checked the correlation between changes in angiographic measurements (perfusion and vascular changes) and changes in various laboratory measurements following urokinase therapy.

There was a small but good correlation for the vascular changes, but less so using data from lung scanning. There was a reasonable negative correlation for the pulmonary arterial pressure and the right atrial pressure. There was little correlation between angiographic improvement and systemic pO_2, cardiac index, fibrinogen, plasminogen and whole blood and euglobulin lysis times.

We also found that patients with low levels of plasminogen, fibrinogen and platelets before treatment tended to bleed more during therapy. There was definite evidence of disseminated intravascular coagulation and some of the patients died.

Doran: Our results confirm Mr. Cotton's findings, though we have used electrical stimulation of the calf muscle, which prevents the fall off in axial blood flow during operation. As Browse and Negus (1970) also have shown, using the radioactive fibrinogen technique, electrical stimulation reduces the incidence of deep vein thrombosis.

Mansfield: One of the factors concerned in the aetiology of major venous thrombosis is external compression on the vein wall. This has been demonstrated to be present in 16 out of our series of 81 patients with iliofemoral venous thrombosis. When significant compression is present streptokinase cannot be expected to restore the vessel to normal, nor indeed can a conventional thrombectomy. We believe that accurate localisation of compression can be made by using the Fogarty balloon catheter filled with opaque medium and observed on the image intensifier. The common compression sites

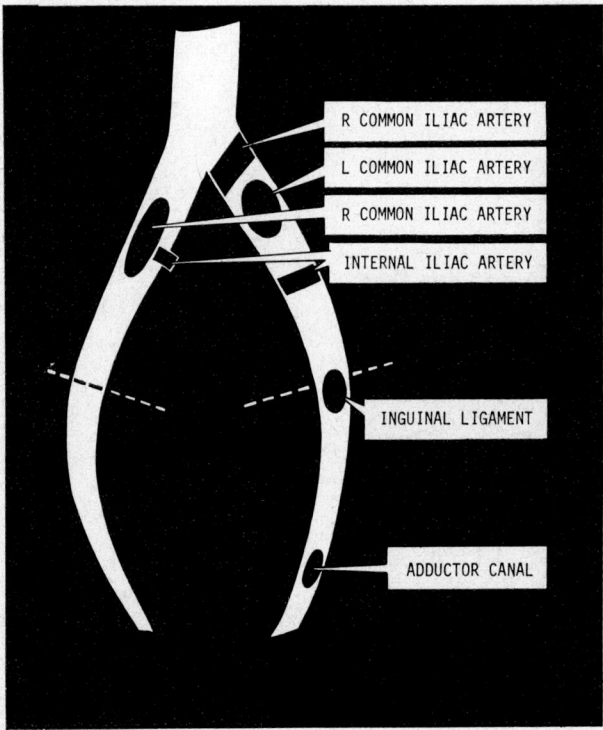

FIG. 20.1. Compression areas in the venous system.

are illustrated in Fig. 20.1 but in addition compression from an unsuspected tumour may sometimes occur. It is our policy to explore and correct such areas of compression except in the case of the right common iliac artery compressing the left common iliac vein.

Howe: Your comments are supported by the long-standing observation that thrombosis is more likely on the left than on the right.

Kakkar: Data assembled by Browse and Negus (1970) suggest there is little difference in incidence between the two sides.

Mansfield: We have had more left-sided thrombosis, but the cause s not just the iliac compression syndrome.

Negus: It should be remembered that, although there is no difference in the left and right incidence of calf vein thrombosis (Browse and Negus, 1970), there is a strong left-sided preponderance of upper femoral and iliac vein thrombosis. This is related to anatomical anomalies at the mouth of the left common iliac vein (Negus et al., 1968).

Sherry: If thrombolytic therapy is to be useful in acute pulmonary embolism, it will be restricted primarily to patients with massive embolism and haemodynamic changes. Therefore it is important to know how quickly thrombolysis can restore normal pulmonary blood flow.

This aspect was not included in the first phase of the urokinase pulmonary embolism trial. However, some workers made sequential studies and were able to demonstrate significant changes as early as two hours—this being the earliest that measurements were taken.

The second phase of our pulmonary embolism trial includes serial measurements. In the streptokinase studies, were observations made early?—this is important in defining the most effective regimen.

Cullum: We have data on two patients only who have received streptokinase and could find no haemodynamic difference.

Sherry: My concern is to develop an optimal therapeutic regimen; then other regimens can be compared with it. There will always be a place for embolectomy; there also will be indications for the use of lytic agents.

Duckert: Professor Widmer's 73 cases can yield more information on the role of thrombus age. There was 94 per cent success with one-day old thrombi, 51 per cent on the second day and 45 per cent on the third. Between the sixth and ninth days the success rate rose to 80 per cent.

These findings correlate with the hypothesis advanced by Gottlob et al. (1971), who believe that clot retraction on the second and third days results in expulsion of serum. On the sixth day, plasma containing plasminogen diffuses into the thrombus.

We prefer the determination of the tolerance to a standard dosage, even the lowest one with 250,000 i.u. as an initial dose, since 68 per cent of our successes were obtained with a lower initial dose. Moreover, the maintenance dose was less than 100,000 i.u. per hour in many instances. We believe that patients with a high tolerance to streptokinase sometimes may have less good results because the high tolerance reflects in some of these patients a low level of plasminogen.

Howe: Dr. Thomas is confident in using anticoagulants, yet many reports show a high incidence of complications. We also get bleeding and have difficulty with control and believe that anticoagulant therapy should never be instituted without venographic proof of thrombosis.

Thomas: Anticoagulant drugs, if used properly and with due attention to recognised contra-indications, have an acceptable incidence of haemorrhagic complications. In the United States pulmonary embolism trial, the incidence of complications in the patients treated with heparin was considerably less than in those given urokinase.

Howe: Would Professor Sherry agree that there is also a quite severe incidence of bleeding with streptokinase therapy?

Sherry: There is a risk of bleeding with streptokinase, probably greater than with heparin. Moreover, the risk of bleeding is enhanced by invasive procedures. In the myocardial infarction trials using streptokinase in several hundreds of patients, but where invasive procedures were kept to a minimum, significant bleeding was not a major problem.

Howe: Why was it thought, in the United States pulmonary embolism trial, that thrombolysis with urokinase was superior? Although the radiographic changes were better, the mortality in the two groups was similar and the morbidity in the urokinase group was greater.

Sasahara: In the study, patients had pulmonary artery catheters, cut-downs and repeated arterial punctures; these invasive procedures invite bleeding, and would not be undertaken in routine clinical use. Spontaneous haemorrhage was similar in frequency in the two groups but was inclined to be more severe in the patients treated with urokinase. Since the mortality in treated pulmonary embolism is relatively low, no real difference in mortality was expected in this relatively small series. A much larger series which is planned will be required before any differences can be shown if indeed there are any. My initial impression is, from perusal of the causes of death, that there will be less mortality with thrombolytic therapy.

Kakkar: Among our 40 patients, 10 bled; four had minor bleeding and six major—though we expected four of these to bleed. One was a young girl with deep vein thrombosis and massive pulmonary embolism—her menstrual period was increased greatly. Another patient bled from the large raw area following radical vulvectomy and a third, who already was bleeding a little from her vagina, following a myomectomy for fibroids, bled more heavily.

We continued treatment in the patients who suffered only minor bleeding, but with the major bleeds, we stopped the infusion, neutralised the circulating activator and gave fresh blood.

In these patients, the vascular bed is not intact. In another 18 patients with an intact vascular bed, there was no bleeding.

Fletcher: Both streptokinase therapy and urokinase therapy are highly dose-dependent. It is possible to administer effective thrombolytic therapy with very little disturbance to the coagulation mechanism, though more monitoring is needed.

Sharp: When is the surgical wound safe for thrombolytic therapy?

Howe: There is no rigid rule; we would not consider a mastectomy safe until about 10 days, whereas an appendicectomy might be safe at five days. The patient with a vulvectomy bled at 9 or 10 days.

REFERENCES

BROWSE, N. L. and NEGUS, D. (1970) *Brit. med. J.*, **3,** 615.
NEGUS, D. *et al.* (1968) *Brit. J. Surg.*, **55,** 369.

Index

Aetiology of thromboembolism, 16, 230-231
  factors, 16
  lithotomy position, 136
  venous blood flow in, 56, 57
  venous stasis in, 160
Age
  as factor in thromboembolism, 16
  of thrombus, 232
  thrombosis and, 136
Ancistrodon rhodostoma, 165
Ancrod,
  compared with streptokinase, 165
  in deep vein thrombosis, 161, 176
  in pulmonary embolism, 165—166
Angiography,
  in pulmonary embolism, 212, 220, 227, 230
    relation to blood pressure, 214, 219
Ante-partum studies of deep vein thrombosis, 132
Anticoagulant therapy, 229
  basis of, 19
  bleeding in, 156
  compared with dextran, 157
  complications, 166, 233
  hypercoagulability and, 20
  in myocardial infarction, 119, 120, 148, 149
  prophylactic use, 155-156
Antithrombin III, 2, 20
  assay of, 51
  inhibitor levels and, 50
  role of, 21
Antithrombotic treatment, indications, 14
Aorto-iliac occlusion, treatment, 147
Arterial embolism,
  compared with venous, 15
  treatment with streptokinase, 147

Arteriography in pulmonary embolism, 184, 189
Aspirin,
  combined with heparin, dangers of, 163
  effect on prostaglandins, 159
  in prevention of thromboembolism, 158-160
Bleeding,
  in anticoagulant therapy, 156
  in heparin therapy, 163
  in streptokinase therapy, 146, 150, 174, 192, 233
  in urokinase therapy, 205, 233
Blood, venous thromboembolism and, 2-12
Blood groups, thromboembolism and, 17, 137
Blood pressure, relation to angiography in pulmonary embolism, 214, 219

Calf muscles,
  electrical stimulation, 72-73, 80-81
Cardiac arrest in pulmonary embolism, 214
Cardiorespiratory arrest in pulmonary embolism, 206
Cerebral haemorrhage, 207
Cerebrovascular thrombosis, diagnosis, 53
Chromatography,
  of fibrinogen, 26
  use in detection of post-operative thrombophlebitis, 31-34
Coagulation,
  endotoxin as trigger, 22
  initiation of, 22
Coagulation factors,
  during pregnancy, 19
  post-operative, 3
  responsible for thrombosis, 19

Complement,
  activation of, 22
Contraceptive pill,
  thromboembolism and, 17, 35–38, 137
Coronary care unit,
  use of ^{125}I-fibrinogen test in, 118–121
Coumarin drugs,
  evaluation, 15
Cryofibrinogen formation, 21

Deep vein thrombosis,
See also Venous thromboembolism
  antepartum, 132–133
  assessment of progress, 171–172
  diagnosis, 126, 131, 135, 169, 178
  See also under tests
    by Doppler ultrasound, 89–99
    by isotopes, 101–115
    ^{125}I-fibrinogen test, 171, 175
    problems, 111
  fibrinogen degradation products in, 173
  incidence, 131, 136
    in orthopaedic patients, 109
    in surgical patients, 108
  in fractures of femoral neck, 123–128
  in myocardial infarction, 13, 110
  in obstetical and gynaecological patients, 109, 131–138
  in orthopaedic patients, 109, 123–128
  in prostatectomy, 121–123
  in urological patients, 109
  lithotomy position and, 136
  localization of site, 128
  phlebography in, 140, 173
  post-operative,
    effect of foot pedalling, 62
    incidence, 97
    intermittent leg compression and, 66
    prevention of, 56
  postpartum, 133
  prevention,
    by electrical stimulation, 70, 73–74, 80–84, 87, 139, 230
Deep vein thrombosis,
  prevention,
    by leg compression, 70
    by leg exercises, 70
  radiography in, 171
  site of origin, 70, 74–77, 84

Deep vein thrombosis,
  soleal veins and, 69
  treatment, 160–161, 175
    ancrod, 161, 165, 176
    comparative results, 176
    heparin, 161, 165
    results of, 172–175
    selection of patients for streptokinase, 170
    side effects of, 174
    streptokinase in, 147, 161, 165, 169–179, 218
Dextran,
  compared with anticoagulants, 157
  in prevention of thromboembolism, 157–158
  post-operative thrombosis and, 5
Diagnosis of thromboembolism, 51, 70–71, 74–77, 169
  See also under methods and individual sites
  importance of, 178
  in obstetric patients, 132
  fibrinogen-fibrin degradation products, 25
  new laboratory tests, 39–47
Dicumarol in prevention of thromboembolism, 158
Dipyridamole,
  prophylactic use, 159
Doppler ultrasound,
  capabilities and limitations, 94–96, 97
  clinical application, 96–97
  correlation with clinical findings, 94
  diagnosis of incompetence of valves by, 93, 95
  diagnosis of occlusion by, 93, 95
  diagnosis of deep vein thrombosis by, 89–99
  interpretation, 93
  method, 89–91

Electrical stimulation in prevention of deep vein thrombosis, 73–74, 80–84, 87, 139
Endotoxin as trigger of coagulation, 22
Enzymes, and emboli formation, 162
European Working Party's Trial of streptokinase, 150

Factor V, 165
Factor VIII, 165

Factor X, 19, 54
  inhibitor of, 20, 21
Factor Xa, 2
Factor XIII, 165
Femoral artery thrombosis,
  treatment, 147
Femoral vein,
  blood flow in, 59
    effect of exercise, 61
    effect of external pressure on,
      60–61
    examination by ultrasound, 91, 93,
      94, 97
Femur,
  fractures,
    deep vein thrombosis following,
      123–128
    prevention of thromboembolism in,
      157, 158
Fibrin,
  impaction in pulmonary vascular
    bed, 50
  nonenzymic formation, 40
Fibrin degradation products, 49, 51, 52,
    169
  detection of, 40
  identification of, 52
  in diagnosis of thromboembolism, 39,
    40
  post-operative, 3, 6
Fibrin monomers, 51, 52
  detection of, 41
  in diagnosis of thromboembolism, 39,
    40
  polymerization of, 42
Fibrinogen,
  chromatography of, 26
  gel elution patterns, 27
  high molecular weight, 26–30
  isotope labelling, 102
  See also ^{125}I-Fibrinogen test
  levels following urokinase therapy,
    199
  molecular weights, 25–30
  pathways of catabolism, 21
  post-operative levels, 6
^{125}I-Fibrinogen test, 2, 53, 85, 117, 132
  accuracy of, 106–107, 132
  advantages and disadvantages of, 112,
    126
  antepartum, 132
  as routine screening procedure, 107,
    112

^{125}I-Fibrinogen test,
  clearance from soleal and tibial veins,
    72, 79–80, 86
  correlation with phlebography, 107,
    110
  correlation with venography, 123,
    125, 127
  development of, 102
  in coronary care unit, 118–121
  in deep vein thrombosis, 50, 171, 173
  in detection of post-operative throm-
    bophlebitis, 31
  in established thrombosis, 110–111
  in orthopaedic patients, 123–128
  in patients with fracture of femur,
    123–128
  in prostatectomy patients, 121–123
  in surgical patients, 107
  post-operative, 10
  postpartum, 133
  procedure, 103–106
  value of, 113, 139
Fibrinogen degradation products,
  identification of, 52
  in deep vein thrombosis, 173
  in venous thromboembolism, 25–38
  molecular weights, 25–30

Gram negative sepsis causing thromboembolism, 16
Gynaecological patients,
  deep vein thrombosis in, 109–110,
    131–138, 157

Haemodynamic measurements
  following urokinase therapy, 202
  in pulmonary embolism, 183, 185,
    186–192
Heart,
  rupture of, 151
Heat stroke, thromboembolic complications, 30
Heparin,
  bleeding complications, 163
  combined with aspirin,
    dangers of, 163
  evaluation, 15
  Factor X inhibitor and, 20
  in deep vein thrombosis, 161, 165
  in prevention of post-operative throm-
    bosis, 53,
  in pulmonary embolism, 161, 182,
    197

INDEX

Heparin,
  mechanism of action, 161
  value of, 229
Hip fractures, 14, 123–128, 157, 158
Hypercoagulability, 11, 13–23
  activator-inhibitor balance in, 50
  assays for, 21
  definition, 19
  diagnosis of, 25, 53
Hypotension, 198, 213

Iliac veins,
  blood flow in, 59
  thrombosis,
    detection of, 112
  venography, 140
Immobilization as factor in thromboembolism, 16
Incidence of thromboembolism, 132, 136
Infection,
  thromboembolism and, 16
Inhibitor, 2
  to Factor X, 20
Isotopes,
  diagnosis of deep vein thrombosis by, 101–115
  in detection of post-operative thrombophlebitis, 30

Kabikinase
  See Streptokinase

Laboratory tests for venous thromboembolism, 39–47
Leg,
  compression of, 70
  electrical stimulation of, 73–74, 80–84, 87, 139, 230
  intermittent compression of, 63–65
  passive exercise of, 70
Leg bandaging, in prevention of thrombosis, 60, 61, 85
Lung scanning in pulmonary embolism, 44, 45, 203
Lysis time, post-operative, 6

Malayan Pit-Viper venom, 165–166
Malignant disease, thromboembolism and, 17
Maternal mortality, 131
Molecular weights of fibrinogen-fibrin degradation products, 25–30

Myocardial infarction, 14
  anticoagulants in, 119, 120, 148, 149
  deep vein thrombosis and, 13, 110
  ^{125}I-fibrinogen test in, 118, 119
  astreptokinase in, 148–151
  urokinase in, 152

National Heart and Lung Institute.
  urokinase pulmonary embolism trial, 195–209

Obstetrics, deep vein thrombosis in, 109, 131–138
Oestrogens, causing thromboembolism, 16
Orthopaedic patients,
  deep vein thrombosis in, 109, 123–128
  prevention of thromboembolism in, 156

Paracoagulation, 40
Phlebography, 229
  correlation with ^{125}I-fibrinogen test, 107, 110
  in deep vein tnrombosis, 107, 140, 173
Plasminogen, post-operative levels, 3
Plasminogen activators, 145, 146, 195
  in lungs, 49
Platelets,
  aggregation, 160
  effect of aspirin on, 159
  effect of heparin on, 162
  prostaglandins in, 162
Platelet adhesiveness, post-operative, 6
Platelet-collagen interaction, 159–160
Platelet count, post-operative, 3, 6
Platelet stickness, post-operative thromboembolism and, 49
Platelet-thrombin interaction, 163
Plethysmography, impedance, 140
Polycythemia vera, thrombosis in, 22
Popliteal veins, examination by ultrasound, 92, 93, 94
Post-operative thromboembolism, 3, 5, 6
  diagnosis, 51
  platelet stickness in, 49
  prevention by heparin, 53
  detection by isotopes, 30
Post-phlebitic syndrome, 114, 139
  prevention with streptokinase, 178
Pregnancy, coagulation factors in, 19

INDEX

Prevention of thromboembolism,
  anticoagulant drugs, 155–156
  aspirin, 158–160
  electrical stimulation, 70, 73–74, 80–84, 87, 139, 230
  foot pedalling, 62–63
  leg compression, 63–65, 70
  passive leg exercises, 70
  with dextran, 157–158
  bandaging in, 60, 61, 85
Prostaglandins, in platelets, 162
  synthesis of, 159
Prostatectomy,
  deep vein thrombosis in, 121–123
Pulmonary angiography,
  in pulmonary embolism, 199
Pulmonary artery obstruction,
  experimental, 223
Pulmonary blood flow, 220
Pulmonary embolectomy in pulmonary embolism, 148, 212–221
  disadvantages of, 216
  mortality, 207, 215, 216, 227
  operative approach, 225
  results, 213
  selection of patients, 212
  technique, 213, 225
Pulmonary embolism, 13, 114, 126, 139
  ancrod in, 165–166
  angiography in, 199, 212, 220, 227, 230
  arteriography in, 184, 189
  cardiac arrest in, 214
  cardiorespiratory arrest in, 206
  central venous pressure in, 225
  choice of treatment, 182–183
  contraceptive pills and, 35–38
  criteria, 14
  diagnosis, 101, 224, 225
  embolectomy in, 212–221
    mortality, 215, 227
    results, 213
  embolectomy in,
    selection of patients, 212
    technique, 225
  haemodynamic findings,
    post-treatment, 185, 186–192
    pre-treatment, 183
  heparin in, 161, 182, 197
  high molecular weight fibrinogen in, 30
  incidence, 101, 131

Pulmonary embolism,
  lung scanning, 203
  mortality, 13
  natural history, 181
  post-operative, 6
  predisposing factors, 224
  prevention, 158–159
  prognosis, 139
  recurrence of, 206
  relation of angiography to blood pressure, 214, 219
  relation to venous thrombosis, 15
  right ventricular systolic pressure in, 202
  serial dilution protamine sulphate test in, 44
  shock in, 152, 207, 219
  streptokinase in, 148, 164, 181–193, 213, 216
    complications, 192
    mortality, 216
  surgical treatment, 148, 223–227
  See also under Pulmonary embolectomy
  symptoms, 224
  treatment, 166
    results of, 185
    thrombolytic, 164
  urokinase in, 151, 195–209, 230, 232, 233
    complications, 204
    dosage, 197
    haemodynamic measurements, 202
    results of treatment, 207, 233
Pulmonary resistance, total, 185, 186, 187
Pulmonary systolic pressure, 183, 185, 186
Pulmonary vascular bed, fibrin impaction in, 50
Pyrexia in streptokinase therapy, 174, 177, 192

Schwartzman reactions, 16
Serial dilution protamine sulphate test, 40, 52
  clinical experience, 44
  technique, 41
Serum hepatitis following ^{125}I-fibrinogen test, 113
Shock,
  in myocardial infarction, 150
  in pulmonary embolism, 152, 207, 219

Sickle cell disease, 22
Sodium diatrizoate, clearance from tibial and soleal veins, 71–72, 77–79, 85, 86
Soleal veins,
  deep vein thrombosis and, 58, 69
  ^{125}I-fibrinogen clearance from, 72, 79–80, 86
  sodium diatrizoate clearance from, 71–72, 77–79, 85, 86
Staphylococcal clumping test, 44–45
Streptokinase, 145–151, 229
  administration of, 170–171
  antigenicity of, 145, 195
  bleeding following, 166, 174, 192, 233
  compared with ancrod, 165
  complications, 150, 192
  disadvantages of, 177
  dosage, 146, 182, 232
  European Working Party's trial, 150
  hazards of treatment, 146
  in arterial thromboembolism, 147
  in deep vein thrombosis, 147, 161, 169–179, 219
    assessment of progress, 171–172
    results, 172–175
    selection of patients, 170
  in myocardial infarction, 148–151
  in pulmonary embolism, 148, 164, 181–193
    haemodynamic findings, 183, 185, 186–192
    results, 185
  injection into thrombus, 176
  in pulmonary embolism, 213, 216
    mortality, 216
  mortality, 150
  other drugs used with, 171
  pyrexia following, 174, 177, 192
  selection of patients, 219
  side effects, 174
  site of action, 196
  technique of therapy, 182
  valvular function following, 178
Surgery,
  ^{125}I-Fibrinogen clearance test during, 72, 79–80, 86
  incidence of deep vein thrombosis in, 108
  measurement of venous blood flow during, 59–60
  passive exercise during, 61–62
Surgical operations,
  hypercoagulability following, 11
  thrombosis following
  See Post-operative thrombosis

Thrombin time during streptokinase therapy, 146
Thrombolytic therapy,
  justification for, 144, 152
  of pulmonary embolism, 164
  value of, 144
Thrombus,
  age effects, 232
  factors involved in formation, 2
  injection of streptokinase in, 176
  resolution, 144, 152, 197, 207
Tibial veins,
  examination by ultrasound, 92
  ^{125}I-Fibrinogen clearance from, 72, 79–80, 86
  sodium diatrizoate clearance from, 71–72, 77–79, 85, 86
Tranexamic acid, 174

Ultrasound, Doppler
See Doppler Ultrasound
Urokinase, 151–152
  bleeding from, 233
  complications of treatment, 166, 204
  dosage of, 197
  fibrinolytic activity and, 199
  in deep vein thrombosis, 233
  in myocardial infarction, 152
  in pulmonary embolism, 195, 230, 232, 233
    complications, 204
    dosage, 197
    haemodynamic measurements, 202
    results, 207, 233
  site of action, 196
Urokinase-Pulmonary Embolism Trial, 151, 164, 195
Urokinase-Streptokinase Pulmonary Embolism Trial, 152
Urological patients,
  deep vein thrombosis in, 109

Valvular function following streptokinase therapy, 178
Venography, 140
  correlation with ^{125}I-fibrinogen test, 123, 125, 127

Venography,
    detecting deep vein thrombosis, 70, 74–77
    disadvantages, 126
Venous blood flow,
See also Venous stasis
    detection by Doppler ultrasound, 90
    dynamics of, 56
    effect of intermittent leg compression, 63–65
    effect of passive exercise, 61–62
    measurement during surgery, 59–60
    thrombosis and, 56, 57
Venous embolism, compared with arterial, 15
Venous occlusion, 93
    detection by ultrasound, 91, 93, 95
Venous pressure in pulmonary embolism, 225
Venous stasis, 85, 161
See also Venous blood flow
    deep vein thrombosis and, 57, 69
    prevention by electrical stimulation, 72–73, 80–81
    reduction of, 70
    role in thromboembolism, 160

Venous system,
    compression areas, 231
Venous thromboembolism,
See also Deep vein thrombosis
    anatomical localization of, 58–59
    contraceptive pills and, 17
    drug treatment, 155–167
    fibrinogen-fibrin degradation products in, 25–38
    in orthopaedic surgery, 156
    laboratory tests for, 39–47
    mortality, 15
    prevention of, 56
    relation to pulmonary embolism, 15
    serial dilution protamine sulphate test in, 40, 46
    treatment, 160–161
Venous valve incompetence,
    diagnosis, 91, 93, 95
Ventricular systolic pressure in pulmonary embolism, 202

Warfarin, in prevention of thromboembolism, 157